PSYCHOLOGY LIBRARY EDITIONS:
EMOTION

Volume 9

ADOLESCENCE, AFFECT AND HEALTH

ADOLESCENCE, AFFECT AND HEALTH

DONNA SPRUIJT-METZ

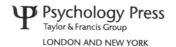

Psychology Press
Taylor & Francis Group
LONDON AND NEW YORK

First published in 1999

This edition first published in 2015
by Psychology Press
27 Church Road, Hove BN3 2FA

and by Psychology Press
711 Third Avenue, New York, NY 10017

Psychology Press is an imprint of the Taylor & Francis Group, an informa business

British Library Cataloguing in Publication Data
A catalogue record for this book is available from the British Library

ISBN: 978-1-84872-780-9 (Set)
eISBN: 978-1-315-73911-3 (Set)
ISBN: 978-1-138-80617-7 (Volume 9)
eISBN: 978-1-315-75180-1 (Volume 9)

Publisher's Note
The publisher has gone to great lengths to ensure the quality of this reprint but points out that some imperfections in the original copies may be apparent.

Disclaimer
The publisher has made every effort to trace copyright holders and would welcome correspondence from those they have been unable to trace.

Adolescence, affect and health

Donna Spruijt-Metz, PhD

Rossier School of Education, University of Southern California

Department of Medical Ethics and the Philosophy of Medicine, Vrije Universiteit, Amsterdam

Netherlands Institute of Mental Health and Addiction, Trimbos-institut

published for

The European Association for Research on Adolescence

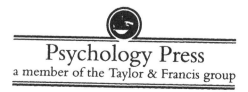

Psychology Press
a member of the Taylor & Francis group

Psychology Press Ltd
27 Church Road
Hove
East Sussex, BN3 2FA
UK

British Library Cataloguing in Publication Data

A catalogue record for this book is available from the British Library

    ISBN 0-86377-518-7 (hbk)
    ISSN 1466-4801 (Studies in Adolescent Development)

Cover design by Jim Wilkie
Typeset by Facing Pages, Southwick, West Sussex
Printed and bound in the United Kingdom by Biddles, Guildford and King's Lynn

For our daughter, Mishala Rebecca
"...And you shall be a blessing..."

Contents

Series preface

At a popular level, adolescence and adolescents are often presented in largely negative terms. Attention tends to focus on features such as awkward and unruly social behaviour, adolescent gangs and their violent, anti-social activities, teenage pregnancy, drug-taking, etc. Such characteristics are portrayed as if they are typical of what adolescents do and accordingly, as a justification for regarding adolescence as a problem period of development.

For much of the 20th century, this popular picture was supported by books and other publications which presented adolescence as a period of "storm and stress". Adolescence was seen as a period of turbulence, inner turmoil and confusion, characterised by conflicts with parents and other authority figures. For psycho-analytic thinkers, for example, conflict was regarded as a normal aspect of adolescence and its failure to appear as an indication of some form of developmental problem.

In the last three decades of the 20th century important changes in this perspective began to emerge. Psychologists began to question the "storm and stress" perspective and to provide evidence that this pattern was neither a typical nor a necessary part of adolescence. Parallel with this, a less problem-centred approach to thinking about adolescence began to emerge: an approach which emphasised the processes of change and adjustment which young people undergo in responding to the varied tasks and transitions with which they are confronted. An increasing number of books and articles on adolescence began to appear and these differed markedly from earlier publications in emphasis and orientation. In contrast to the clinical-descriptive approach which had been prevalent for much of the century, this new work was based on an empirical approach and focused upon a variety of specific aspects of adolescent development. Such publications stimulated further interest in adolescence as an area of study and in doing so, started a process which led to the emergence of research on adolescence as one of the most active fields of developmental research of the present day. As a result, discussion of topics relating to adolescence has become a prominent feature of developmental conferences and scientific journals in North America, Europe and elsewhere.

The presence of this series, "Studies in Adolescent Development" is a further reflection of the increased interest in adolescence as an area of study. While adolescence as a research area is well served by a range of academic journals, more detailed accounts of specific areas of study within this period of development are more difficult to find. The present series aims to change this state of affairs by providing a range of books, each of which deals in depth with a topic of contemporary interest within the field of adolescent development. Each book is written by an expert on a specific aspect of adolescence and sets out to give a clear picture of the sort of research activity which is currently serving to extend the boundaries of our knowledge and understanding of the field.

The series is itself the outcome of co-operation between Psychology Press and the European Association for Research on Adolescence. The latter is an organisation which aims to promote and safeguard high quality fundamental and applied research on all aspects of adolescent development. Each book in the series can be seen as a further step in the fulfilment of this aim. The Association is grateful to Psychology Press for all that it has done to develop and promote the series and for assisting the Association to extend knowledge of current research on adolescent development.

Sandy Jackson,
Series editor
June 1999

Preface

When I was first offered the opportunity to work on this project, there was nothing on paper, no description, and no plan. What became my project was merely part of a larger idea that lived entirely in the mind of my friend and colleague, Jan M. Broekman. In the years that I have had the privilege of working with him, he gained my deep respect for his speed and agility in grasping ideas from various disciplines and putting them to work. I want to thank him for the freedom he gave me to fill in his philosophical ideas with my methodological and positivistic ways of doing things, and for the inspiration he always seemed to have in ready supply.

Many other colleagues deserve my heartfelt thanks for their contributions to this research. I especially want to thank Johan Hoogstraten for his fine ideas and methodological input, and Willem Koops for his guidance and inspiration. My husband and colleague Rob Spruijt is an artistic methodologist and statistician. His fingerprints are all over this book and I am very grateful for his continuing involvement in my work. He is second author on Chapters 6 and 9, and furnished valuable advice for many of the other chapters.

Thanks are due to Evert van Leeuwen at the Department of Philosophy and Medical Ethics at the Vrije Universiteit Amsterdam, where most of this book was written, for the intellectual and academic freedom, camaraderie, support, and mutual respect. Annette Kalf provided much needed medical expertise, and was observer for the interviews.

Several other people deserve special thanks for their help and participation. Ruud Emous and the people at the LGVO in Utrecht were invaluable. For their assistance in the organisation of the focus group interviews, I would like to thank Erna Klein Ikkink, Peter Molenaar and Joke Velzen. Capi Wever was kind enough to serve as an observer on some of the interviews. My thanks also go to Ellen de Boer, Ester

Kappert, Ybeline Walinga, Ingrid Wigard, and Wieke de Vent, the psychology students who assisted in the third phase of the research. I am grateful to Loek Pijls, who provided invaluable advice on nutrition and nutritionists for the fourth phase of the study, and Katharina Meerum Terwogt-Kouwenhoven, who corrected my Dutch in the lesson material. Beebs van Riessen, who did the graphic design and DTP for the lesson materials, was (as always) a pleasure to work with. My thanks go to the team (and my cousin) at the Printing Press in Carson, California, for producing the artwork for the book. Thanks also go to the psychology students who assisted in the fourth phase of the research: Carine Aberson, Anna Diepraam, Lies Vereecke, Sandra van Dijk, Taco Reus, and Sascha Ripken.

This book never would have seen the day without Sandy Jackson, President of the European Association for Research on Adolescence. I am deeply indebted to him for making publication possible. Thanks are also due to the four reviewers who so carefully went over my work. Their invaluable advice helped to improve the original manuscript immeasurably. I am grateful to the people at Psychology Press who have made the publication process an easy one.

None of this research would have been possible without the participants. My sincere gratitude goes to all the adolescents and teachers who participated in the interviews, surveys, and the effect study, to the teachers who were willing to test the lesson materials, to the school administrators who allowed us to conduct our research in their schools, to the doctors, nutritionists and dietists who filled in the arduous questionnaire to provide up-to-date information for the lesson materials, and to all those participants and colleagues who gave their time to this project.

Mishala, our daughter, didn't really help with the research, although her intimate relationship with sweets did serve as an inspiration for further research. Her presence brightened my days and kept my feet on the ground.

Donna Spruijt-Metz

February 1999

Los Angeles, California

Introduction

Why do some adolescents undertake some healthy behaviours? Why do they undertake risky behaviours, even when they 'know better'? According to one very eloquent adolescent girl, it has to do with making one's own rules instead of blindly following the rules that others lay down for you. It has to do with learning to make your own choices, exercising your own will. Perhaps there is a fine balance between breaking perceived rules and developing autonomy. She explained that breaking some rules made you a better person, while breaking other rules made you a lesser person.

Many health habits are developed and consolidated during adolescence, and the health habits that are developed during adolescence will continue to influence health throughout the life span (Cobb, 1998; Hurrelmann, 1990; Jessor, 1984). As adolescents begin to claim their independence, to make career choices, and to form mature relationships, they also encounter and experiment with many healthy and risky behaviours (Coleman, & Hendry, 1990; Hurrelmann, & Lösel, 1990). At the same time, adolescents are beginning to be able to reason hypothetically, to conceive of causes and effects in terms of pluralistic causality and multiple outcomes, and to distinguish appearance from reality (Cobb, 1992; Coleman, & Hendry, 1990; Craig, 1983; Gilligan, 1988; Kohlberg, 1984). Given relevant information and guidance, adolescents are thus ready to understand the often complex information about health, to relate that information to their own behaviour, and to base their choices on this understanding. Much adolescent health research and education is directed at high-profile risk behaviours, such as smoking, drinking, drug abuse and unsafe sex. While there is no question that these important threats to adolescent health demand continued attention in adolescent health research and education, the relative lack of research on everyday health-related behaviours, such as eating and sleeping habits, forms a major lacuna in the literature. And although research is rapidly accumulating in the field of adolescent health, adolescent health education is often fragmented and ineffective (Froman, & Owen, 1991). Taken together, these findings suggest that adolescence is a particularly important period for relevant health education concerning everyday health-related behaviours. These are some of the observations that sparked the research described in this book.

The main objective of the research reported here was to develop and evaluate relevant and effective health education materials for Dutch adolescents concerning everyday health-related behaviours. In order to ensure that the materials would be relevant, information was needed on what these adolescents generally do in terms of health-related behaviour, and which areas of health they themselves consider to be relevant or important for health education. The adolescents' general knowledge, values, attitudes, beliefs, and feelings concerning health also needed to be explored. To ensure that the materials would be effective, the major determinants of health-related behaviours in the target population had to be established, and methods for influencing these behaviours had to be explored. To accomplish these goals, the research was carried out in four phases: theoretical, qualitative, quantitative, and applied.

THE THEORETICAL PHASE: BUILDING A THEORETICAL BACKGROUND

The theoretical phase of the research is reported in the first three chapters of this book. In Chapter 1, the multidisciplinary nature of health education research is emphasised. Because many different disciplines participate in health education research, all with their own jargon, it is important to periodically agree upon shared definitions for the central terminology. Definitions for health, health education, health promotion, and health-related behaviour to be used for the duration of the present research are offered in this chapter. Adolescence is also defined, and the interrelationships between this period of life and general health are established. Because educating youth in health-related matters is a big responsibility, we feel that it is important to keep the pitfalls and limitations of the undertaking in mind. To this end, Chapter 2 reviews some ethical issues involved in adolescent health research and education. In Chapter 3, 14 theories on the determinants of health-related behaviour are reviewed in order to form an impression of their usefulness for adolescent health research and education.

THE QUALITATIVE PHASE: LETTING THE SUBJECTS SPEAK

Chapter 4 and Chapter 5 report on the qualitative phase of the research. Because much information concerning the target population was needed, and because much of the research in the fields of adolescent health and health education has been conducted using samples made up of American college students, it was essential to consult the target group as an integral part of the project. Chapter 4 reports results of a partially open questionnaire on health-related behaviours and several aspects of physical and psychological well-being. Chapter 5 reports on a series of focus group interviews conducted with the target group.

THE QUANTITATIVE PHASE: FORMULATING THEORY

The results of the theoretical and descriptive phases of the research were used to formulate hypotheses and research questions for the survey questionnaires used in the quantitative phase of the research. The results are reported in Chapters 6, 7, and 8. In order to understand what motivates adolescents to undertake behaviours, the hierarchy of their major concerns and the place of health within this hierarchy required study. In Chapter 6, the general concerns of the target group were explored, their major health complaints were inventoried, and the relationship between worrying and health in the population was explored. In Chapter 7, everyday health and risk behaviours were inventoried. The conclusions from the theoretical phase and the data from the focus group interviews resulted in the formulations of a series of hypotheses, or mini-theory. The theory was that adolescents tended to imbue health-related behaviours with meanings, and that salient meanings of health-related behaviours in turn became determinants of those behaviours. In Chapter 8, these hypotheses were tested for a number of everyday health-related behaviours.

THE APPLIED PHASE: CHANGING ADOLESCENT HEALTH-RELATED BEHAVIOUR

Often, the trajectory of a research programme will end at the quantitative phase. Once a construct has been shown to successfully predict behaviour (once a correlational relationship has been found), it is frequently assumed that the construct in question is therefore a determinant of that behaviour (a cause-and-effect relationship is assumed). However, applied research and programme evaluations have repeatedly shown that this is not always the case (Chapter 3). Good predictors of behaviour do not always prove to be useful in the field. Can meanings of behaviour actually be manipulated, and will changes in meanings lead to changes in behaviour? To answer these questions, a final, applied phase of the research was undertaken. Chapter 9 reports the development, implementation, and evaluation of an intervention based on the theory of meanings of behaviour.

PART ONE

Building a theoretical background

CHAPTER ONE

Adolescent health education and research: Defining terms

INTRODUCTION

In the 1970s, discussions of behaviours such as drinking, smoking, drug abuse, and promiscuous sex could be found under the heading of *anti-social behaviours* (Marsh, Rosser, & Harré, 1978). Nearer the new millennium, discussions of the same behaviours are usually found under the heading of *health-related behaviours* (Cobb, 1992; Glanz, Lewis, & Rimer, 1997). This illustrates not only the increasing medicalisation of our lives, but also the need to update the definitions of scientific terminology at more or less regular intervals. Definitions change as knowledge grows. What is meant by the catch-phrase 'Health in the Year 2000' (US Department of Health and Human Services, 1995)? What is healthy behaviour, what is the difference between health promotion and health education, and how are these concepts related? Research is continuously modifying our understanding of adolescence, of health, of health education, and of health education research. This leads to subtle shifts in the meanings and scope of the concepts used to speak about what we know. Therefore, the central constructs need to be chosen and defined to ensure that we are all speaking the same language *before* we embark upon an in-depth discussion of adolescent health and health education. Scientific fields tend to gather tacit assumptions like stones gather moss as the research (and the jargon) expand. These assumptions are often overlooked at the onset of an analysis, or (often erroneously) presumed to be understood, shared, and axiomatic. These tacit assumptions need to be unearthed, interpreted, and re-examined in the light of new findings *before* analysis is undertaken. While any definition of terms or elucidation of assumptions is by nature of temporary validity, they may nonetheless be considered prerequisites to research. This first chapter is what might be called an epistemological analysis of the constructs and assumptions in adolescent health and health education research (Broekman, pers. comm.). To carry out this analysis, the chapter proceeds in two sections, moving from the subject matter to the subjects themselves. First we look at the three main concepts used in this book. These are health behaviour, health, and health education. Next, we take a look at adolescents, the subjects of the research presented here. How is adolescence defined? Is there a unique relationship between adolescence and our three main concepts? If so, what is the nature of the relationship between adolescence, health behaviour, health, and health education?

HEALTH-RELATED BEHAVIOUR

Perhaps the central construct in health education and research is 'health-related behaviour'. Two central *assumptions* in health education and research are (1) the existence of a causal link between behaviour and health and (2) that behaviour (and consequently health) can be regulated through health education. Health-related behaviour is the main subject of research and the ultimate target of interventions. Although the classification as *education* implies a focus on dissemination of information, the primary goal of health education is to improve health by effecting changes in health-related behaviour (Glanz et al., 1997). Health-related behaviour is often partitioned into two categories: *risk* behaviour (or health-risk behaviour) and *health* behaviour (or preventive health behaviour) (Donovan, Jessor, & Costa, 1993; Terre, Ghiselli, Taloney, & DeSouza, 1992). *Risk* behaviours are expected to endanger health and *health* behaviours are expected to enhance health.

The broad definition of health from the Ottawa Charter (World Health Organization, 1986) leads to broad categories of health and risk behaviours. These are behaviours that may affect physical health, mental health, social well-being, or any combination thereof. Health-related behaviour may incur proximal or distal health effects, or a combination of the two. Risk behaviours can refer to behaviours that bear obvious and immediate health consequences, such as driving under the influence of alcohol. Risk behaviours can also refer to behaviours that compromise future health. For instance, inadequate calcium intake in childhood and adolescence increases chances of osteoporosis later in life. Some risk behaviours, such as dietary habits contributing to obesity, have both short-term and long-term consequences for health. Risk behaviours can jeopardise mental and physical health or social well-being now and in the future, just as health behaviours can enhance these immediately or prospectively. Note that assigning any particular behaviour to the category of 'health' or 'risk' behaviour is dependent upon the state-of-the-art of medical and health-related knowledge and research. The healthy or risky nature of many behaviours is subject to lack of consensus and (occasionally abrupt) changes in status or credibility (see Box 1.1: Controversy on health-related behaviour).

By far the most satisfying conclusion to this paragraph would be an exhaustive list of health-related behaviours, which could then be neatly and conclusively

> **Box 1.1: Controversy on health-related behaviour**
>
> A case in point concerning the stability of our knowledge on health-related behaviour is the controversy surrounding possible health benefits and risks linked to consumption of the various types of dietary fats. Cardiovascular disease causes 34% of all deaths among adults in the United States (Centers for Disease Control, 1998). These deaths are often premature and preventable through behaviour modification (World Health Organization, 1998). Precisely which behaviours are healthy and which are risky remains the issue. Valid, well-designed research has repeatedly shown that high dietary fat intake and obesity are cardiovascular health risks. Diets low in fat, especially in saturated fats, have been endorsed by many of the leading nutrition experts and heart health organisations in the Western world (Sizer, & Whitney, 1997). However, some researchers claim that it is more important to increase the intake of unsaturated fats than to decrease the intake of saturated fats (Oliver, 1997; Sacks, & Willet, 1991). Findings have also suggested that while the percentage of overweight and obese children is on the rise, and while these children are at substantial health risk, reduction of dietary fat could lead to important risk of unsatisfactory intakes of fat-soluble vitamins (Vobecky, Vobecky, & Normand, 1995). But when the American Heart Association changed their dietary recommendations to reflect some of this new research, some scientists came out strongly against these changes. After careful review of the literature, they were convinced that the recommendation which the American Heart Association had given for over 30 years was still the only responsible prescription for cardiovascular health in the light of existing research (Heyden, 1994). (This advice was: limit the fat intake to 30% of total calories, with 10% derived from polyunsaturated fatty acids, 10% from monounsaturated fatty acids, and 10% from saturated fatty acids.) Finally, some research groups concluded after carefully controlled studies that the interpretation of the effect of diet, dietary fat or a specific fatty acid on the development of chronic disease is extremely complex (Mutanen, 1997).

organised into healthy and risky behaviours in the following two paragraphs. However, ongoing research and changes in paradigms continually add to our knowledge and transform our way of interpreting what we know (Spruijt-Metz, 1998a). Therefore, a definitive list cannot be compiled, and we cannot systematically amalgamate information from all the health web sites, wellness newsletters, and research findings into one final product. What remains is a careful examination of the *concepts* used in this book, without delineation of precise content. The examples used are equally subject to controversy and changes in status as our understanding of health-related behaviour evolves.

Health behaviour

The concept of health behaviour has enjoyed a longstanding conceptual discourse in the literature. Kasl and Cobb (1966) defined health behaviour as any activity undertaken by people who consider themselves to be healthy, such as regular check-ups. In this definition, health behaviour is undertaken for the purpose of preventing disease or detecting it in an asymptomatic state. Kasl and Cobb differentiated health behaviour from illness behaviour. Illness behaviour was defined as behaviour undertaken by those who perceive themselves as 'ill' in order to reduce or remove complaints. Harris and Guten (as quoted in Kendall & Turk, 1984) included symptomatic individuals in their concept of 'health-protective behaviours', and incorporated health-promoting, health-maintaining, and disease preventing behaviours into this concept. Taylor (1986) simply defines health behaviour as behaviour undertaken to enhance or maintain health. This definition fits with a broad definition of health, and includes behaviours with both proximal and distal effects on physical, mental, and social well-being. Incorporated into this conceptualisation of health behaviour are activities such as proper diet, safe sex, and regular exercise. Gochman (1982) recognised that overt behaviour is not the only direct influence on health, and included reportable or measurable feeling states and mental events in his definition of health. His comprehensive vision of health behaviour included (Gochman, 1982, p. 169): "those personal attributes such as beliefs, expectations, motives, values, perceptions, and other cognitive elements; personality characteristics, including affective and emotional states and traits; and overt behaviour patterns, actions and habits that relate to health maintenance, to health restoration, and to health improvement". This definition includes determinants of behaviour as well as behaviour itself. It must therefore be used with the utmost caution in order to avoid the confounding of dependent and independent variables (Cook, & Campbell, 1979; Whitehead, 1994). While this broad definition of health behaviour is to be applauded conceptually, the inclusion of personal attributes makes it difficult to separate cause from effect. For instance, it is possible that a positive outlook on life influences health, perhaps by mediating our motivation to carry out healthy behaviours. It is equally plausible that physical health contributes to a positive outlook on life, which in turn might facilitate our ability or motivation to engage in healthy behaviours. Along these lines, research into explanatory styles (or how people explain events) has shown that people with an optimistic explanatory style tend to experience better health (Peterson, & Bossio, 1991; Seligman, 1995). Optimists also tend to undertake more healthy behaviours. Another finding is that children can be 'trained' in optimism (Seligman, Reivich, Jaycox, & Gillham, 1995). This illustrates the difficulties one can run into when trying to formulate conceptually satisfying as well as researchable definitions of healthy behaviour: the dependent and independent variables here are firmly intertwined, as they are in Gochman's definition. Does optimism lead to health, or does health lead to optimism?

Glanz, Lewis, and Rimer (1997, p. 9), cite a powerful definition of health behaviour: "health behaviour refers to the actions of individuals, groups, and organisations, and to those actions' determinants, correlates, and consequences, including social change, policy development and implementation, improved coping skills, and enhanced quality of life". This definition places the individual firmly in a social context. It extends the concept of health behaviour out towards care for the environment, social and political involvement, religious activities, and the like. It also includes behaviour as well as determinants of behaviour, and requires the same cautious use as the above definitions.

A final word on health behaviour must be accorded to the champions of enjoyment. This group of researchers is challenging the standard division between healthy and risky behaviours, which they see as rigid, moralistic, and counterproductive. They are amassing some interesting research on the health-enhancing aspects of enjoyment. This includes findings on the positive influences of some behaviours that have come to be considered health risks. According to some very distinguished scientists, behaviours such as drinking as much coffee and alcohol as you want, and eating as much chocolate as you feel like may have salutary effects on health, provided that you thoroughly enjoy it (Associates for Research into the Science of Enjoyment (ARISE), 1999; Snel, 1996)!

Health behaviour as understood in this book is a synthesis of several approaches. Concepts have been borrowed from various disciplines, including psychology, medicine, medical sociology, and behavioural medicine. The challenge of scientifically responsible inclusion of personal attributes into a broad definition of health behaviour is accepted. Medically related behaviours such as regular check-ups and participation in screening programmes are taken into account. Activities that improve our society or environment are included. The possibility that dominant ideas concerning healthy behaviours might be rigid, moralistic, and counterproductive is kept in mind. In this context, health behaviour is defined as any overt behaviour or personal attribute that is considered to contribute to distal or proximal enhancement, maintenance, and/or restoration of physical, mental, and social well-being, and/or to (distal or proximal) disease prevention.

Risk behaviour

While risk behaviour is frequently a hot topic in adolescent health behaviour research, it has not enjoyed as much fundamental discussion as health behaviour, and it is implicitly assumed that while we might not know what is good for us, we certainly know what is bad for us. The concept of risk behaviour applies to overt risky behaviour, but also to the absence of health-enhancing behaviours. Health risks can be incurred by the individual, or be present in the environment or in situational factors. According to Jessor (1984), the concept of risk behaviour reflects the balance between health-compromising and health-enhancing activities undertaken. In the area of adolescent health research, Jessor and his group researched a subset of risk behaviours, which they term 'problem behaviours'. They have amassed evidence showing that these behaviours, including smoking, drinking, alcohol and drug abuse, and precocious sexual activity constitute a syndrome of interrelated behaviours (Jessor, 1984, 1991). There is evidence that one risk behaviour leads to another, which lends empirical support to the concept of a coherent risky adolescent lifestyle. Comparable support for the existence of coherent *healthy* adolescent lifestyles, however, has not been found (Spruijt-Metz, 1996; Spruijt-Metz & Spruijt, 1996).

Risk behaviour is understood in this book in the same broad context as health behaviour, and the set of qualifying remarks made at the conclusion of the preceding paragraph hold for this one as well. Placed in this context, any overt behaviour or personal attribute that jeopardises distal or proximal physical, mental, or social well-being, or promotes disease, is considered to be 'risk behaviour'.

Transgressional vs. everyday health-related behaviour

Besides the distinction between health and risk behaviour, another distinction has been made in the attempt to classify and research health-related behaviours. This distinction is between behaviours that involve transgressions of societal norms and those which do not (Donovan, Jessor, & Costa, 1991; Donovan et al., 1993; Elliot, 1993; Jessor, 1984). Transgressional behaviours are morally laden behaviours, such as sex-related behaviours and substance abuse. These behaviours depart from the regulatory norms of adult society. Transgressional risk behaviours are socially negatively qualified behaviours, forcefully condemned by adults, media, institutions and so forth (Donovan et al., 1991; Spruijt-Metz, & Spruijt, 1996). They represent serious violations of social norms, and sometimes also violation of legal norms (Elliot, 1993). Transgressional health behaviours are often defined as the absence or renunciation of trangressional risk behaviours. However, some health behaviours are transgressional in their own right. Safe sex between 10-year-olds might be a good example. On the other hand, everyday health and risk behaviours are not ensconced in a stringent moral network. These are common behaviours that influence health, such as eating patterns and sleeping habits.

Everyday behaviours have received less attention than the transgressional type of behaviours, with the notable exceptions of diet, exercise, and seat belt use (Parr, 1988; Stacy, Bentler, & Flay, 1994; Tappe, Duda, & Menges-Ehrnwald, 1990). Adolescent health research and education is often aimed at curtailing physical risks incurred by transgressional behaviours. However, the definition of health in the Ottawa Charter stresses the importance of health enhancement before the fact, and conceives of health as a feeling of overall well-being, including mental and social well-being as well as physical well-being. From this point of view, common, everyday behaviours form the basis for present and future health and well-being, and deserve detailed study (Cobb, 1998; Jessor, 1984). The protective influence of religious activities on health during adolescence has been documented (Jessor, 1984; Resnick et al., 1997). Social skills (Bijstra, van der Kooi, & van der Molen, 1993; Perry, & Kelder, 1992) and choosing clothes appropriate to season and climate (Spruijt-Metz, & Spruijt, 1996) are two more examples of everyday health behaviours. Explanatory style and optimism have been identified as correlates of physical well-being (Peterson, 1995). Explanatory style and optimism are considered behaviours (rather than traits or characteristics) because they are subject to change through training and health education (Seligman, 1995). In line with this reasoning, pessimism would be considered an everyday risk behaviour, as would poor dietary habits. In general, too little is known about the mechanisms at work in these all-important everyday health-related behaviours (there are exceptions, such as those mentioned above). Certainly, the last word has not been spoken on how to effectively promote and maintain everyday healthy behaviours in adolescent populations. In keeping with Seligman's push for a positive psychology, there is a need to balance psychology's focus on repairing damage and avoiding risk with a psychology that can promote health and well-being before the fact (Sleek, 1998). This demands the study of normal development, human strength, buffering agents, and factors that contribute to survival and resilience. In the area of health behaviour and education, this calls for an emphasis on everyday behaviours, especially everyday health behaviours.

From the preceding analysis, four categories of health-related behaviours can be distilled: (1) transgressional risk behaviours such as smoking and drinking, (2) transgressional health behaviours which are often interpreted as the renunciation of (or abstention from) transgressional risk behaviours, such as quitting a drug habit, (3) everyday risk behaviours such as inadequate exercise, and (4) everyday health behaviours such as sufficient sleep (Spruijt-Metz, 1996).

We have seen how shifts can occur in our categorisation of behaviours as 'healthy' or 'risky' as progress in research influences our knowledge and understanding. Other factors can also lead to shifts in categorisation, such as cultural norms, principles of ethics and incumbent moral systems. Similarly, shifts between the categories of 'transgressional' and 'everyday' will occur. These changes in view are spurred only in part by science and research. Changes in legislation can also lead to changes in categorisation of behaviour as 'transgressional' or 'everyday'. Morals and ethics change, and these changes effect our views on human behaviour (Beauchamp, & Childress, 1989). As morals and ethics shift, so will the view on what is to be considered 'transgressional'. In the field of adolescent health, age and development also influence our views on the healthiness and acceptability of behaviour. Behaviour that might be considered risky as well as transgressional for a child of 10, such as sexual intercourse, becomes normative for a late adolescent nearing 20 years of age.

Having said this, the 2 × 2 table of behaviours in Table 1.1 provides a useful framework for the study of adolescent health, if the permeability of the boundaries is kept in mind. The focus of this book is on health education and research

TABLE 1.1

Four categories of health-related behaviours

Category	Transgressional	Everyday
Risky	Transgressional risk behaviours	Everyday risk behaviours
Healthy	Transgressional health behaviours	Everyday health behaviours

pertaining to the third and fourth categories during a specific period of life, taken together as everyday health-related behaviour during adolescence.

HEALTH

Needless to say, *health* is one of the central constructs in health education and research. In the preceding section, the word appeared 114 times! It is such a common word, that we are tempted to read over it without questioning its meaning. Perhaps this is why health is often left undefined in health education research. Sometimes definition is avoided due to the incredible intricacy of the concept. A sound background in philosophy would be required to understand and synthesise the voluminous literature generated in the ongoing discussion on the definition of health (Black, Boswell, Gray, Murphy, & Popay, 1984; Caplan, Tristram Engelhardt, & McCartney, 1981; Moreillon, 1992; Shiloh, & Waiser, 1991). Different cultures, different age groups, different professionals, and different people with different life experiences will define health differently (Bouter, pers. comm.; Wallander & Siegel, 1995; Wilson, Rodrigue, & Taylor, 1997). It is therefore essential to state clearly how health is to be defined, although it may seem alternately redundant or alienating. Within the context of this book, health is understood in accordance with the definition provided in the constitution of the World Health Organization (WHO), adopted in 1946, and endorsed in the Ottawa Charter for Health Promotion (World Health Organization, 1986, p. iii). The WHO defines health as "a state of complete physical, mental and social well-being". This definition is important to the research presented here for three reasons. In the first place, health is conceived of as more than the absence of disease. This pushes the goals of health education past prevention by incorporating the promotion of health-enhancing behaviours, alongside the more traditional prevention of impaired health and health risks. In the second place, the broad scope of the definition implies an expansion of the terrain of health-related policy and research by pulling in behaviours and situations relating not only to physical, but also to mental and social well-being. In doing so, it echoes a pattern of cultural values. In the third place, the definition cited here offers basic criteria for development of health research and education, and a sound basis for criticism: physical, mental and social aspects must be taken into account.

HEALTH EDUCATION

Definitions

The Ottawa Charter, from which the above definition of health was quoted, pertains to health promotion. Health promotion offers comprehensive approaches to the enhancement of public health. The US Department of Health and Human Services defines health promotion as "any combination of health education and related organisational, political, and economic interventions designed to facilitate behavioural health" (US Department of Health and Human Services, 1980). The Ottawa Charter defines health promotion as "the process of enabling people to increase control over, and to improve, their health" (World Health Organization, 1986. p. iii). Green and Kreuter (1991) define health promotion as "the combination of educational and environmental support for actions and conditions of living conducive to health". Health promotion is, thus, an umbrella term which subsumes activities undertaken on the community or aggregate level, the interpersonal or group level, and the individual level. It includes goals related to environmental, social, political, organisational, policy, and economic interventions, as well as to individual behaviour change.

According to the definitions of health promotion cited above, health education is one of the central components of health promotion. The body of research on health education and health behaviour has increased exponentially over the last two and a half decades, and health education has gained recognition as a valuable resource for meeting public health objectives (Glanz et al., 1997). The Joint Committee on Health Education Terminology report (1990, p.103) defines health education as the "continuum of learning which enables people, as individuals and as members of social structures, to voluntarily make decisions, modify behaviours, and change social conditions in ways which are health enhancing". Green, Kreuter, Deeds, and Partridge (as quoted in McKenzie & Lurs, 1993) define health education as "any combination of learning experiences designed to facilitate voluntary adaptations of behaviour conducive to health". Some researchers prefer to use the terms 'health promotion' and 'health education' interchangeably (Glanz et al., 1997). Others find it valuable to make a distinction between the two (Green, & Kreuter, 1991; McKenzie, & Lurs, 1993). In this book, the distinction is considered essential for an in-depth understanding of the field. The concept of health promotion delineates a large-scale operation that may be undertaken simultaneously on many levels (including individual, group, community, political, national). Health education is an integral part of health promotion. However, health education as understood here can be undertaken independently of large-scale health promotion efforts. This kind of smaller-scale health education project might be initiated at only one or two levels (usually personal and group/school and/or family). Health *education* alone is usually cheaper, quicker and easier to implement than health promotion offensives. The broader thrust of health *promotion* programmes may contribute to (long-term) effectiveness (Green, & Kreuter, 1991).

Assumptions

Alongside these formal definitions, several assumptions are involved in the tenet of health education. One is the assumption that health problems can be identified and understood. Another is the assumption that appropriate intervention programmes and prevention strategies can be developed to deal with the identified health problems. A third assumption is that people can be taught to assume responsibility for their health and that this will in turn change their health behaviours and lifestyles (McKenzie, & Lurs, 1993).

These assumptions, however, are not always met: The difficulties involved in the identification and understanding of health problems are illustrated by the ongoing controversy surrounding low cholesterol diets and by the lack of consensus concerning the effects of monosaccharides on health and behaviour (Sizer, & Whitney, 1997). While it cannot be denied that there have been major changes in health-related behaviours in many western nations over the past two decades (Glanz et al., 1997), the extent to which these changes can be attributed to health education is still under debate (Liedekerken, Jonkers, de Haes, Kok, & Saan, 1990). For instance, smoking has been reduced in several nations (Centers for Disease Control, 1998; Canadian Council for Tobacco Control, 1998; Cancer Society of New Zealand, 1998) and cardiovascular health has improved world-wide (World Health Organization, 1998). Many factors influence these changes. The literature testifies to the fact that some credit must go to effective health education programmes (Glanz et al., 1997; Perry, & Kelder, 1992; Tones, & Tilford, 1994). However, this same literature shows that effective programmes are difficult to design, and that the scope and determinants of effectiveness are equally difficult to evaluate.

The assumption that people can be taught to take responsibility for their health and that this will in turn change their behaviour, has proven one of the most difficult to meet. Changing behaviour is difficult for several reasons. *Habit* is strong and resistant to interventions (Triandis, 1977). *Knowledge* alone is not enough to influence behaviour (Parcel, 1984). Also, there must be some kind of *motivation* for or interest in change before behaviour will be changed (Kelly, Zyzanske, & Almegano, 1991). And should behaviour change be accomplished, it is difficult to *maintain* (Becker, 1990).

The above mentioned assumptions culminate in two final assumptions: the assumption that health status can be changed, which is directly related to the assumption that changes in individual and societal health-related behaviour will affect an individual's health status positively. The central objectives of health education invariably focus on health-related behaviour modification and change, i.e. the reduction of risk behaviours and the enhancement of health behaviours. Health-related behaviour is at the heart of every definition of health education and is the principal dependent variable in research on the effectiveness of health education interventions. Few of the studies on the effectiveness of health education programmes actually monitor projected changes in health. Instead, they evaluate changes in target behaviours. As Glanz et al. (1997, p. 9) put it: "Positive informed changes in health behaviour are typically the ultimate aims of health promotion and education programs; if behaviours change but health is not subsequently improved, the result is a paradox that must be resolved by examining other issues...".

The fact that the several assumptions inherent in health education and research are not always met need not necessarily be an obstacle, as long as they are clearly recognised. In any scientific undertaking, implicit assumptions tend to blur observation and threaten validity (Cook, & Campbell, 1979; Hacking, 1983). It is, therefore, important to keep assumptions explicit and to be aware of the extent to which they are in place at any point in time along the path of planning, creating, implementing, and evaluating health education programmes. An essential step here is to carefully define the target group and address tacit assumptions about that group. This book is about health research and education for adolescents. But to whom are we referring when we say 'adolescents'? What *do* we know about adolescents and adolescence? Can we tease out differences between solid knowledge and insubstantial assumptions made about this group? Is health education relevant for various adolescent populations, and if so why?

ADOLESCENCE AND HEALTH

Most adolescents accord little thought to health-related matters (Elliot, 1993; Spruijt-Metz, & Spruijt, 1997), and why should they? Adolescence is generally a time of radiant health and well being, and the approaching years bear the promise of the greatest physical strength to be achieved during the life span. Yet research has shown that the period of adolescence is especially relevant for health and health education (Cobb, 1992; Cobb, 1998; Janz, & Becker, 1984; Jessor, 1991, 1993; Millstein, Petersen, & Nightingale, 1993b; Resnick, & Rozensky, 1996; Wilson et al., 1997a). To illustrate this point, research on all four categories of health-related behaviour will be cited in the following paragraphs. This is in part necessary to give a fuller picture of the impact of behaviour on adolescent health. It is also unavoidable because, as stated above, the bulk of research on health-related behaviour in adolescence is on (transgressional) risk behaviours. Even when research is done on both healthy and risky behaviours, results are often reported in the negative: the emphasis is on risk and avoidance of risk rather than on health behaviours and their promotion (Box 1.2: Defining terms: Teasing out categories of behaviour). Having said this, the results of the research reported below reflect the urgent need for effective and relevant adolescent health education.

Researchers at the Adolescent Health Program at the University of Minnesota and the Carolina Population Center at the University of North Carolina at Chapel Hill (Resnick et al., 1997, p. 823) agree that "The main threats to adolescents' health are the risk behaviours they choose." They arrived at this conclusion using data gathered in the National Longitudinal Study of Adolescent Health (Add health). This conclusion attests to the fact that a great deal of the mortality and morbidity that occurs during adolescence is behaviour-based, and is thus preventable under the assumption that behaviour can be modified or changed.

According to the Centers for Disease Control, only four behaviour-based causes account for nearly three-quarters of all mortality and a great deal of morbidity in American youth between 5 and 24 years of age. These are motor vehicle crashes

Box 1.2: Defining terms: Teasing out categories of behaviour

The research being done in such projects as the YRBSS (Youth Risk Behaviour Survey System), the National Longitudinal Study of Adolescent Health (Add Health), and the Monitoring the Future (MTF) on risk behaviour in adolescence is important and necessary. However, the main focus of much of this research tends to be on (transgressional) risk behaviour. This can make it difficult to tease out information on everyday health-related behaviour from existing sources. Data are notably lacking on the healthy behaviours, their determinants, maintenance, and long-term effects. A good example of emphasis on risk is the 1995 Youth Risk Behaviour Survey. This is a large-scale national study involving hundreds of high schools across the United States. The YRBSS surveyed six types of risk behaviours, which were broken down into five subcategories (Centers for Disease Control, 1998). These are reproduced here in full:

A. Unintentional and Intentional Injuries
1. Rarely or never used safety belts
2. Rode with a drinking driver during past month
3. Carried a weapon during past month
4. Were in a physical fight during past year
5. Attempted suicide during past year

B. Alcohol and Other Drug Use
1. Drank alcohol during past month
2. Reported episodic heavy drinking during past month
3. Used marijuana during past month
4. Ever injected illegal drugs
5. Ever sniffed or inhaled intoxicating substances

C. Sexual Behaviours
1. Ever had sexual intercourse
2. Ever had four or more sex partners
3. Had sexual intercourse during past three months
4. Did not use a condom during last sexual intercourse
5. Did not use birth control pills during last sexual intercourse

D. Tobacco Use
1. Ever smoked cigarettes
2. Smoked cigarettes during past month
3. Smoked cigarettes on 20 or more days during past month
4. Used smokeless tobacco during past month
5. Not asked proof of age for purchase of cigarettes

E. Dietary Behaviours
1. Ate <5 servings of fruits and vegetables yesterday
2. Ate >2 servings of high-fat foods yesterday
3. Thought they were overweight
4. Were attempting weight loss
5. Took laxatives or vomited to lose or maintain weight during past month

F. Physical Activity
1. Did not participate in vigorous physical activity
2. Did not participate in moderate physical activity

3. Were not enrolled in physical education class
4. Did not attend physical education class daily
5. Exercised <20 minutes in an average physical education class

The YRBSS does include several everyday risk behaviours (A 1, B 1, C 1–5 [depending on the age group], E 1–4, and F 1–5). However, in order to tease out statistics on everyday health behaviours from this study, one would have to look at the mirror images of the statistics on these categories. However, this study is not designed to look at healthy behaviours, buffering effects, or factors that contribute to resilience. Therefore, merely 'flipping' the statistics will not yield (content) valid results (Cook, & Campbell, 1979).

The Add Health Study, now ongoing in the United States, offers useful data on a broad spectrum of both everyday and transgressional health behaviours, although the emphasis remains on risk (the credo of the project is 'reducing the risk') (Blum, & Rinehart, 1997). This extensive study boasts tens of thousands of participants, over 2000 variables, is longitudinal, and includes data gathered from adolescents, their parents, schools and friends (Bearman, Jones, & Udry, 1997). Needless to say, a database this size will cover a great deal of territory, including variables from all four categories of health-related behaviour. An example of results from the Add Health Study in the area of everyday health-related behaviours: those who took part in religious activities participated in fewer everyday and transgressional risk behaviours (Resnick et al., 1997). An entire generation of research remains to be done with this incredibly rich database.

What is 'behaviour' exactly?

We tend to think of traits, personality, and characteristics as being fairly stable constructs, which are not under voluntary control. In other words, these are considered to be aspects of individuals or systems that cannot be influenced, taught, learned, or modified easily. An example: Parent–family connectedness and school connectedness were found to be protective against a broad spectrum of risk behaviours in the Add Health Study (Resnick et al., 1997). Is connectedness a behaviour? Or is it a trait or characteristic of a particular family, a specific school? 'Connectedness' as conceptualised in the study could be viewed as involving a series of behaviours that can, to some extent, be modified. As soon as there is evidence that modification is possible, constructs tend to inch away from the 'trait' or 'characteristic' categories and towards the area of 'behaviour'. A case in point is the discussion on optimism. Optimism, once considered a trait, has moved closer to classification as a behaviour since it has been shown that it can be taught and modified (see Seligman et al., 1995).

(29% of all deaths), homicide (20%), suicide (12%) and preventable injuries (11%). (Centers for Disease Control, 1989).

Running a close fifth are sexually transmitted diseases and unintended pregnancy (Centers for Disease Control, 1998). Youth Indicators, 1996, published by the US Department of Education, National Center for Education Statistics, also maintain that mortality of persons 15 to 24 years of age is largely attributable to behavioural causes (Snyder, & Shafer, 1996). They add a sixth major cause of death and morbidity to the above list: cancer and (heart) disease. Researchers have narrowed down the risk behaviours causing a great deal of this grief to six types: accident and suicide-related behaviours, alcohol and drug use, sexual behaviour, tobacco use, dietary behaviours, and physical activity. These behaviours are currently being monitored by the YRBSS (Youth Risk Behaviour Surveillance System) (Centers for Disease Control, 1998).

In The Netherlands, a full 42% of the deaths registered in 1996 for 10–19-year-olds was due to accidents (83% of these were traffic accidents) (Hoogenboezem, 1998). In the *Life in the 21ˢᵗ Century* report recently released by the World Health Organization, adolescence is conceptualised as a transition from childhood to adulthood marked by potentially deadly 'rites of passage'. According to the WHO, the main threats to adolescent health in the 21st century will be violence, delinquency, drugs, alcohol, motor accidents and sexual hazards (such as HIV and unwanted pregnancy) (World Health Organization, 1998).

Aside from the overwhelming evidence on preventable morbidity and death through risk behaviour *during* adolescence, health-related behaviours undertaken during adolescence will influence *future* health. Many health-related behaviours are initiated, tried out, explored, and learned during adolescence. While different determinants of health-related behaviour are championed by the many extant theories in the field, there is wide consensus and ample empirical support for *past behaviour* as one of the major determinants of *future behaviour* (Ajzen, & Madden, 1986; Bentler, & Speckart, 1979; Triandis, 1977). In other words, behaviour that is familiar is likely to be repeated. Habits and tastes, which are acquired and consolidated during adolescence, will affect adult health (Cobb, 1998; Millstein et al., 1993b; Tappe et al., 1990; Wilson, Nicholson, & Krishnamoorthy, 1997a). Many behaviours that are assets to health in later life, such an inclination for regular exercise or a preference for healthy foods, are developed in childhood and adolescence (Telama, Yang, Laasko, & Viikari, 1997). Conversely, many behaviours that involve prospective health risks, such as becoming accustomed to a poor diet or practising unsafe sex, also appear to develop during adolescence. These habits and predilections that emerge during adolescence predict both behaviour and health in later life (Petridou et al., 1997). Findings on osteoporosis illustrate 'hidden' influences of behaviour during adolescence on future health. Risk varies with ethnicity, but most women in the Western world are at risk for osteoporosis as the life expectancy is pushed upwards. The lifetime risk of fragility fracture for a 50-year-old Caucasian woman is about 40 per cent (Chapuy, & Meunier, 1995). There is consensus in the medical world that prevention of this debilitating disease begins with nutrition, adequate calcium intake, and regular exercise during childhood and adolescence (Kulak, & Bilezikian, 1998; Masi, & Bilezikian, 1997).

The convergence of health and adolescence can best be illustrated through a description of the nature of adolescence, as it is understood throughout this book. The theoretical framework within which adolescence will be defined here is referred to as the lifespan approach. The lifespan approach to adolescence (Cobb, 1998; Coleman, & Hendry, 1990; Jessor, 1984) is particularly well suited to adolescent health research for three reasons. In the first place, it integrates several perspectives on adolescence, including chronological, historical, biological, psychological and developmental, cognitive and moral, anthropological, sociological, and legal criteria. In the second place, the lifespan approach stresses both continuity and change in development. In the third place, the lifespan approach is inherently multidisciplinary.

Facets of adolescence and links to health

Chronological age. Chronological age is an assessable marker for any particular period of life. Adolescence is often equated with 'teens' and 'teen-age'. Some authors differentiate between early (10 to 15 years of age) and late adolescence (15 to 19 years of age) (Cobb, 1998; Millstein, Petersen, & Nightingale, 1993a). Others differentiate between early (11–14 years of age), middle (15–17 years of age), and late (18–20 years of age) (Crockett, & Peterson, 1993). In this book, the early/late differentiation is used. Primary developmental issues and experiences of early adolescents differ markedly from those of late adolescents (Cobb, 1992; Coleman, & Hendry, 1990; Marcia, 1994). Early and late adolescents have also been shown to differ in health-related behaviours, which supports the relevance of this chronological differentiation for health behaviour research (Spruijt-Metz, & Spruijt, 1996). However, although chronological differentiation is a handy heuristic, it has many disadvantages and can be misleading. Adolescents demonstrate substantial variability on many measures of development. In other words, individual differences in development are large and chronological differentiation must be used with care, and preferably along with other perspectives. One of the main advantages of the lifespan approach to development is that it synthesises many different perspectives on adolescence.

The historical perspective. The historical perspective on adolescence recognises that the texture of adolescence changes as society changes. Even the length of adolescence is affected by societal changes. Improved nutrition and childcare have contributed to the secular trend, which refers to the fact that puberty begins earlier and children grow faster than in the past. Improved conditions and medical care have also extended life expectancy. We live longer, and the period referred to as adolescence has stretched along with life expectancies. The generally accepted age of onset of early adolescence has crept forward, and late adolescence has been attenuated. Education has been prolonged, commitment is often postponed, and the period that Erikson (1963) referred to as 'moratorium' has been extended. The speed of social change, the existence of pluralistic value systems, and the rapid accumulation of knowledge have made the Western world less accessible for children and young people (Koops, 1990). This has contributed to the prolongation of adolescence. The changing face of adolescence can be linked to health and health education in many ways. One link, is the fact that policies in public health, health insurance, and health care do not always reflect the changing needs of adolescent populations (Levenson, Pfefferbaum, & Morrow, 1987; Moreillon, 1992).

Biological criteria. Biological criteria, such as the onset of puberty and the growth spurt, are often used to define the beginning of early adolescence. The onset of puberty and the growth spurt, which occur simultaneously, are regarded as separate but related biological phenomena. Puberty is marked by the onset of sexual maturation, involving many physical changes, including hormonal changes, the addition of subcutaneous fat for girls and muscle mass for boys, development of secondary gender characteristics, the onset of menses for the girls and the growth of testes and penis for the boys. During the growth spurt, which usually peaks during early adolescence for girls and at the beginning of late adolescence for boys, 20% of adult height and up to 50% of adult weight is added. Forty-five per cent of skeletal growth takes place throughout early and late adolescence. These physical changes place special demands on the body, and give rise to special nutritional needs (Parr, 1988; Pipes, & Trahms, 1993; Sizer, & Whitney, 1997; Voorlichting voor de Voeding, 1993; Voedingsraad, 1986). There are two inescapable facts about diet and adolescence. The first is that diet is extremely important for optimal growth and health during adolescence. The second is that a healthy diet during adolescence reduces the risk of chronic diseases in later life (Contento, & Michela, 1998). However, adolescents often meet increased needs for minerals (such as calcium and iron) and vitamins (such as C and B6) with erratic eating habits and junk food (Cobb, 1992; Contento, & Michela, 1998; Parr, 1988; Pipes, & Trahms, 1993; Spruijt-Metz, 1995; Voorlichting voor de Voeding, 1993).

Psychosocial development. The developmental perspective on adolescence, included in the lifespan approach, proposes that the convergence of physical maturation with changing personal and social expectations confronts adolescents with new developmental tasks (Havinghurst, 1972). These tasks are representations of the culture's definition of normal development at different points of life (Cobb, 1998). Early adolescence is identified with changing sex roles, with working towards more autonomous relationship with parents, and with working towards more mature relationships with peers. According to many theorists, the main developmental task in this period is gaining autonomy, defined as becoming independent and taking responsibility for one's actions (Cobb, 1998; Craig, 1983; Erikson, 1963).

While the early adolescent works toward autonomy, the late adolescent works toward identity formation. Identity has been defined as the creation of an integrated self and the consolidation of the changes that accompany autonomy into a mature personality structure (Coleman, & Hendry, 1990; Erikson, 1963; Havinghurst, 1972). This involves attaining emotional independence, exploring sex roles and integrating sexuality into their relationships, forming mature relationships, preparing for adult work roles and a career, and assuming social responsibility. Late adolescents thus deal with changes in their relationships and take steps toward the commitment that will define their adult social roles (Marcia, 1994). The concept of identity has been explored by many theorists (Cobb, 1998). Erik Erikson (1963) emphasised three domains of identity: sexuality, occupation, and ideology (religious and political beliefs). James Marcia (1994) expanded on Erikson's work and delineated four different identity statuses, or ways by which adolescents arrive at the roles and values that will define their adult identities. Adolescents who explore many possibilities in life and make choices that fit them best are termed *identity achieved*. Those who explore but fail to see the importance of making choices are termed *identity diffused*. Those who explore but are afraid to make choices are said to be in *moratorium* and those who do not explore, but adopt their parents' values without question are labelled *identity foreclosed*. Jane Kroger found that shifting back and forth between identity statuses is to be expected. She also found that an individual's identity status may vary over domains (sexuality, occupation, and ideology) (Cobb, 1998).

The research on identity is extensive and fascinating. It is beyond the scope of this book to give a complete review. However, the processes of achieving autonomy and identity formation are intricately connected to health behaviour and education. Social and personal expectations change during the process of identity formation. More responsibility and independence is given to (or taken by) adolescents as they begin to make their own plans for the future. They often have their own money to spend, and may spend it on commodities such as junk food and cigarettes which pose potential risks to health (Van Asselt & Lanphen, 1990; Spruijt-Metz, 1998; Viet, Baltissen, & Syperda, 1995). Adult controls on health-related behaviours diminish, and this can have adverse effects on behaviour and health. For instance, family supervision of diet becomes more limited during adolescence because food is more frequently purchased independently. This reduction of family influence on eating patterns during adolescence generally has a negative effect on nutrition (De Bourdeaudhuij, 1996, 1997a, 1997b). Peers become more important, and more activities take place outside of the home with less adult supervision (Cobb, 1998; Coleman, & Hendry, 1990). Potentially health-compromising elements such as alcohol, drugs, mopeds, motorcycles, and automobiles become more accessible, and there is more opportunity to try them out in an 'adult-free' environment (Hurrelmann, & Lösel, 1990; Jessor, 1984). Jessor (1984, p. 73) speaks of a new developmental task for adolescents: "namely, the assumption and management of personal responsibility for their own health and social responsibility for the health of others". However, the tasks and changes described here, as well as recent research on the topic, indicate that adolescents are often preoccupied with other, for them more pressing issues, than the effect of their behaviour upon their health and that of others (Spruijt-Metz, & Spruijt, 1997; Chapter 5 of this book).

Cognitive and moral development. Changes in cognitive and moral development are also used to define adolescence within the lifespan approach. Early adolescents know more, reason faster, and remember better than children. They can solve more complicated problems, think on more abstract levels, and understand complex social situations. Late adolescents can conceive of the outcomes of their actions in probabilistic terms. They can conceive of causes and effects in terms of pluralistic causality and multiple outcomes, and progress in the ability to distinguish appearance from reality (Cobb, 1998). The cognitive developments that take place during adolescence have been the subject of much theory. Whichever of the many theories of cognitive development appeals, all converge on abstract thought as the major cognitive development in early adolescence. Many focus on the use of abstract thought to formulate a set of values and an ethical system to guide behaviour during late adolescence (Cobb, 1998; Coleman, & Hendry, 1990; Gilligan, 1988). As adolescents develop the ability to think in terms of multiple causes and effects and to reason hypothetically and abstractly, they become ready to understand the often complex and sometimes inconsistent information about health, and to connect that information to their own actions (Crockett, & Peterson, 1993; Millstein et al., 1993a).

Of course, the higher the value placed upon health, the more motivation there will be to seek out, understand, and act upon health-related information (Lau, Hartman, & Ware, 1986). We are inundated daily with information that may be pertinent to our health by the various media, including popular publications and news media, scientific publications, and the information highway. This information is often difficult to access and evaluate, difficult to understand and incorporate into personal decisions and actions, and of a changeable nature because it is always subject to new research (see Chapter 2). Learning how to take responsibility for one's own health and behaviour becomes a complex activity that demands time and practice, and keeping abreast of the new developments in health technology and policy requires a personal commitment to health. The development of a personal system of beliefs, morals, and values goes hand in hand with cognitive development and identity formation (Cobb, 1998). During this time, personal health will receive a more or less stable place in the hierarchy of the adolescent's value system. While cognitive abilities to understand difficult principles related to health are developing, the value system that will determine the importance of personal health is being formed. The moral fabric is being woven within which many health-related behaviours, such as sexuality and substance use, will be judged (Gilligan, 1988; Kohlberg, 1984). This takes place at a time when, as mentioned above, personal freedoms and responsibilities are increasing and new health-related behaviours are being tried out. Taken together, this means that adolescence may be a particularly significant time for health promotion and health education.

Institutional definitions. The description of adolescence offered here is a normative one. However, the processes involved in physical, cognitive, and social development are subject to tremendous individual differences through genetic, environmental, personal, medical, and many other influences. Moreover, the development of a mature physical apparatus, abstract thought, and social skills proceed unevenly and are often domain specific. Many areas of immaturity may remain (Brown, DiClemente, & Reynolds, 1991; Kroger, 1988). This makes it difficult to establish the exact perimeters. While puberty provides convenient criteria for the onset of adolescence, other criteria are necessary to demarcate its upper boundary (Cobb, 1998; Jessor, 1984). Social criteria, such as completion of secondary school, and legal criteria, such as reaching voting age or an age that is legally defined as adult, are often used for this purpose. In this way, development is viewed in terms of the progress made through various social institutions. From a sociological point of view, adolescents are neither self-sufficient, thus not adults, nor completely dependent, thus not children, and therefore the end of this period is often marked by legal criteria specifying age limits for legal protection. When adolescents come of age legally, their parents are no longer accountable for their actions. They are formally able to make their own decisions. Depending on the particular activity (voting, driving a car, marrying, buying alcohol, dying for one's country) and the particular legal system, adolescents achieve legal autonomy somewhere between 16 and 21 years of age. Responsibility for their health and well-being now belongs formally to the adolescents themselves.

CULTURE, ETHNICITY, AND MINORITY STATUS

Much of the research on adolescents and adolescent health to date has been conducted with middle class, Western, Caucasian (often American) persons between 11–19 years of age. It must be kept in mind that in much of the literature the term 'adolescent' therefore refers to middle class, Western, Caucasian (often American) persons between 11–19 years of age. The emphasis on this group has lead to a dearth of relevant theory and research pertaining to other groups (Jessor, 1993). An upsurge of new research is quickly filling in the gap. We are finding that all of the above mentioned facets of adolescence are subject to cultural differences (Frosch, 1995; Wilson et al., 1997a). This means that findings about health habits studied in one group will not necessarily generalise to another group. Cultural and/or ethnic differences have been found in diet (Wilson et al., 1997b), medical consumption (Netherlands Central Bureau of Statistics, 1992), oral hygiene (Verhips, 1993), substance abuse and violence (Botvin, & Scheier, 1997), physical exercise (Taylor, Beech, & Cummings, 1997), and many more areas of adolescent health, health behaviour, and well-being (Wilson et al., 1997a). For instance, Mexican-Americans eat differently from European Americans (Wilson et al., 1997b), Turkish youths living in the Netherlands eat differently from their native Dutch counterparts (Spruijt-Metz, 1996). Cultural and ethnic differences have also been found in fundamental health-related issues such as the value placed on health and the way in which physical symptoms are experienced and reported (Spruijt-Metz, 1998; Spruijt-Metz, Hoogstraten, & Broekman, 1994). Based on available literature, one could surmise that cultures and ethnic groups differ in many, if not most health-related behaviours. Because habits differ, the same health education interventions will not be relevant for all groups. It is not only differences in health, values on health, and health-related behaviour that dictate the necessity for taking culture and ethnicity into account in health education and research. Cultural and ethnic differences inform nearly every domain relating to health. Differences have been found in how behaviour is interpreted, in biological, social and psychosocial developmental processes, in social resources and intergenerational frameworks, and in socialisation, to name but a few areas (Wilson et al., 1997a). Therefore, culture and ethnicity will influence determinants of behaviour, and must dictate approach, language, and numerous other essential facets in research and intervention design.

Cultural differences in health-related areas are often masked or exacerbated by differences in socio-economic status (SES). This complicates the study of adolescent health and health behaviour, because it is often difficult to ascertain the differential effects. The ethical implications of 'correcting' for culture (and thus claiming differences are attributable to SES), or 'correcting' for SES (and thus claiming the opposite) have been intensely debated (Jackson, & Sellers, 1997). In addition, minority status often goes hand in hand with lower SES. Profound influences of minority (and immigrant) status on health and health-related behaviours have been found throughout the world (Chigier, & Nudelman, 1994; Earls, 1993; Jackson, & Sellers, 1997; Wilson et al., 1997b).

Interactions between culture, ethnicity, low SES, minority status and immigrant status can prove detrimental to health and health behaviour and are, to date, poorly understood (Jackson, & Sellers, 1997). The problems of confounding the effects produced by one of these issues with the effects produced by another in health research and health education are immense, purely on the level of research design and statistical analysis (Klerman, 1993; Mackenbach, 1992; Wilson et al., 1997a; Zola, 1966). Additionally, many heated discussions have taken place between researchers on how to correctly interpret these multiple differences. How do they arise? What is the main source? Is there a main source? Can a simple causal model be drawn? Which effects are attributable to which conditions? The answers chosen to these types of questions have enormous influence on how we proceed in health education and research, and can in turn dictate policy, cash flow, and availability of specific health services. It is therefore essential that both the separate and cumulative effects of minority status, SES, culture and ethnicity be understood and taken into account in adolescent health education and research.

GENDER

Gender differences in health and health behaviour are well documented (Alexander, 1989; Avison, & Mcalpine, 1992; Cohen, Brownell, & Felix, 1990; Pennebaker, 1982; Spruijt-Metz, 1995; Spruijt-Metz, & Spruijt, 1997; Terre et al., 1992). Some examples: in Western society, girls report more health complaints, more health-

Box 1.3: More definitions: Culture, ethnicity, and race

Culture, ethnicity, and *race* can be confusing terms. Their accepted meanings have changed over the years. They mean different things to different people. They have come to bear subtle connotations. The on-line Merriam-Webster Dictionary (1998) gives the following definitions:

Culture: the customary beliefs, social forms, and material traits of a racial, religious, or social group.

Ethnic: of or relating to large groups of people classed according to common racial, national, tribal, religious, linguistic, or cultural origin or background.

Race: a division of mankind possessing traits that are transmissible by descent and sufficient to characterise it as a distinct human type.

The main characteristics in these three definitions are hopelessly intertwined. Therefore, they cannot be differentiated in 'the field'. Adherence to such definitions can lead to misconceptions and just plain sloppy research. Moreover, the usefulness of this kind of race concept in health education and research is debatable. For the duration of this book, I am going to honour the definitions for culture, ethnicity, and race chosen by Jackson, and Sellers (1997). These are:

Culture: "a symbolic vehicle of meaning, including beliefs, ritual practices, art forms and ceremonies, and such informal practices as language, gossip, stories and rituals of daily life" (Jackson, & Sellers, 1997, p. 32)

Ethnicity (ethnic group): "a segment of larger society whose members are thought, by themselves and/or others, to have a common origin and to share important segments of a common culture and who, in addition, participate in shared activities in which the common origin and culture are significant ingredients. Some mixture of language, religion, race and ancestral homeland with its related culture is the defining element. No one by itself [sic] demarcates and ethnic group" (Yinger as quoted by Jackson, & Sellers, 1997, p. 33)

Race: Race is often used as a social construct that represents social, psychological, and possibly biological variables. It is poorly defined, randomly employed, and usually poorly differentiated from minority status, ethnicity, and culture. Jackson and Sellers suggest that the concept of race should be rethought and, in its present form, has no place in the social sciences.

related worries, poorer dietary and exercise habits, and go to the doctor more often. Boys report more smoking, more substance abuse, more unsafe sex, and more violence (Sallis, 1993; Snyder, & Shafer, 1996; Viet et al., 1995). Girls and boys also differ markedly in health-related concerns (Millstein, 1993; Spruijt-Metz, & Spruijt, 1996). The subject of gender differences in health and health-related behaviour is a recurring motif throughout this book. Gender differences are manifested in behaviour, beliefs about health and health-related behaviour, health-related knowledge, and behavioural determinants. Moreover, gender differences interact with culture, ethnicity, minority/immigrant status, and SES to create unique health risks for different groups of adolescents. So, not only are girls at higher risk for eating disorders, for instance, but the risk factor is different over different minority groups (Guthrie, Caldwell, & Hunter, 1997). The relationships between gender and culture/ethnicity can be complex. For instance, while Western girls report more symptoms than their male counterparts, girls from Mediterranean countries such as Turkey and Morocco appear to report fewer symptoms than Turkish and Moroccan boys (Spruijt-Metz et al., 1994). These relationships must be understood in order to create relevant and responsive interventions. Any effort in health research and education must take gender differences into account, right down the line of the entire trajectory through research design, data analysis, intervention development, implementation and evaluation.

ADOLESCENCE: CONTINUITY AND CHANGE

The lifespan perspective stresses both continuity and change in the life cycle. Many of the changes that take place in adolescence have now been discussed. Alongside this change is continuity. There is a personal continuity throughout the life cycle. One and the same person passes through the life cycle, and individuals shape their own development. They are active agents involved in an interactive and ongoing process. The lasting effects of adolescent experience and behaviour on adult health demonstrate this continuity. There are many examples of this continuity. For instance, psychological problems in adolescence have been shown to be good predictors of mental illness (Cobb, 1998; Coleman, & Hendry, 1990). Problem behaviour in adolescence is predictive of problem behaviour in young adulthood (Jessor, 1984, 1991). Obesity in childhood increases risk of obesity or eating disorders in adolescence, which in turn can increase the risk of cardiovascular disease in later years (Cobb, 1998; Parr, 1988; Sizer, & Whitney, 1997). The state of the art in medical knowledge disallows the compilation of a complete inventory of the lasting interactions between adolescent health-related behaviour and adult health.

Besides personal continuity, there is continuity in the issues to be coped with throughout the life cycle. Different periods in life share similar issues, which must be dealt with on different levels at different times in life. Autonomy, for instance, is tremendously important to adolescents, but also to toddlers and to the elderly. While adolescents deal with an upsurge in energy, the middle-aged and elderly must also deal with changes in energy levels. While adolescents are borrowing the keys to the car, the elderly are handing them in as levels of independence fluctuate. Changes in body image must be dealt with at regular intervals throughout life.

It is interesting to note that, in keeping with the principle of continuity, the lifespan perspective does not accept the tenet of normative turmoil during adolescence. There is no empirical support for extra moodiness in adolescence, and little empirical support for the existence of a generation gap. Parents and adolescents have been found to agree on values and attitudes more than adolescents and their peers agree on these same issues (Cobb, 1998; Coleman, & Hendry, 1990; Lau, Quadrel, & Hartman, 1990; Perry, Kelder, & Komro, 1993). Turmoil in adolescence is, just like turmoil in any other phase of life, not the norm. Serious conflict with parents is not a phase to be expected, but a good predictor of young pregnancy, suicide attempts, drug usage, and other health hazards.

ADOLESCENT HEALTH RESEARCH AND EDUCATION: MULTIDISCIPLINARY FIELDS

The definitions given in this chapter illustrate the complexity of the field of adolescent health and health education. This is compounded by the intricacy and diversity of accompanying health-related issues, and demands a broad scope of knowledge and expertise from many areas. Knowledge is needed from clinical, developmental, and health psychology, from anthropology, from methodology and epidemiology, from medical sociology and sociology in general, from economics, and from the field of education. Philosophy and medical ethics offer insight into the foundations, presuppositions and 'a priories' in the various fields, and enforce the need to make ethical orientations explicit. Medical and dental information, results from bioscientific research, information from the areas of nutrition, diet, sport, and exercise science all come together in health education endeavours. This list of disciplines that can contribute to adolescent health research is not meant to be exhaustive, but to be illustrative. Each discipline comes equipped with its own terminology, assumptions, and ideologies. Some converge, some diverge in meaning while using the same vocabulary, and some terminologies are indigenous to specific fields. The difficulty of attaining clear communication between researchers and practitioners in so many fields may be evident, it is compounded when information from many fields is necessary but expertise from only a few is present. While adolescent health research and education is a multidisciplinary problem, providing large scale multidisciplinary teams to supply multidisciplinary answers is often not feasible, and researchers from one field must often assume responsibility for accruing knowledge in another field. In these cases, when relevant specialists are not directly available, their expertise must be accessible and understandable to researchers in related fields through the literature. To further mutual comprehension within the context of research requiring co-operation between such a diversity of fields, the need to clearly and regularly define central concepts cannot be emphasised enough.

During adolescence, many behaviour patterns develop that will affect health throughout the life span. Simultaneously, cognitive and moral developments are taking place that enable adolescents to understand and utilise health-related information. This makes adolescence a prime period for effective and relevant health education. To do it right, central terminology must be periodically redefined and implicit assumptions must be monitored. This is not only because of the multidisciplinary nature of the endeavour, although that does make the need urgent. It also has to do with the continual inundation of new knowledge and information. We are forever amassing new data that in turn change accepted knowledge. These change need to be reflected in health research and education.

CHAPTER TWO

Ethical issues in adolescent health education

INTRODUCTION

There are numerous ethical and moral questions raised in the process of implementing health education aimed at behavioural change (Rouwenhorst, 1977), especially when the target group is comprised of children or adolescents (Stanley, & Sieber, 1992). What right do we have, as health educators, to attempt to influence or manipulate the behaviour of others? This question becomes especially meaningful when we consider that school-age children may become a captive audience to interventions they did not choose. These populations are often not in the position to be able to make an informed choice for or against an intervention. They may not be equipped to understand the ramifications of some health-education programmes. Other related ethical questions also come to the fore. How far can we go in our efforts to influence the behaviours, opinions, attitudes, and choices of children and adolescents? How far *must* we go if available knowledge attests to a need for our endeavour? To what extent do we impinge on freedom of choice? How will our efforts affect development?

Ethical perspectives offer valuable insights into the process and the product of adolescent health education. By including ethical considerations up front, one is forced to recognise and acknowledge one's own values and norms about what is desirable or 'good'. After all, any decision to intervene implies judgements about 'what is' as being insufficient: not good, not enough or not optimal. The decision to intervene implies preconceived ideas about 'what should be'. We are compelled to regard our choices on which behaviours in the area of interest are to be considered normative or dysfunctional as ethical or moral judgements. We must then dredge up and clarify the facts and beliefs upon which we base these distinctions in order to justify our choices. This in turn requires the delineation of perceived differences and similarities between normative, dysfunctional, and optimal development (Danish, 1990).

Up until the present, studies in health psychology and behavioural health have not customarily been evaluated in terms of ethical perspectives. This is perhaps in part due to the undeniable fact that ethical and moral issues tend to raise complex problems for which there are no immediate solutions. What I want to propose here is that the study of ethics will not culminate in a 'cookbook' for the avoidance of and/or solution to ethical dilemmas. Rather, the examination of ethical questions that arise in relation to research and education can serve as constant reminders of issues that must be handled thoughtfully. The considerations presented here are intended to provide a conceptual backdrop for adolescent health education. Problems will be delineated, but may not be 'solved' in the process.

Box 2.1: Ethics as philosophy

To those of us who are not trained in the science of philosophy, the word 'ethics' probably suggests a set of standards or principles by which a group or community decides to regulate its behaviour. These standards are used to determine what is acceptable and what is not. When we think of ethics, we usually think principles to live by, moral standards, guidelines for daily life (Flew, 1984). Ethics as a philosophical endeavour is connected to this everyday understanding of the term. The subject matter remains the same. However, instead of taking systems of beliefs as guidelines for living, the ethicist takes them as objects of study. Ethicists study the fundamental principles and basic concepts at the basis of various systems of moral beliefs and principles.

Within philosophy, ethics is a generic term for various approaches to the study of moral life. Several strategies for dividing the field into meaningful sub-fields have been suggested. The following strategy is extrapolated from Beauchamp and Childress' book (Beauchamp, & Childress, 1989).

1. Normative* ethics: The investigation into content of moral principles and virtues, and their justification in terms of the human condition. To quote Beauchamp and Childress (p. 4), normative ethics is the study of: "which general norms for the guidance and evaluation of conduct are worthy of moral acceptance, and for what reasons?"

2. Applied (or practical) ethics: When we try to work out the implications of ethical theories and moral philosophy for specific areas of conduct and moral judgement, we are engaged in applied or practical ethics. Practical ethics are usually discipline-specific, and address the specific problems, practices and policies of that discipline. An example of practical ethics is bioethics, or medical ethics. It is important to note that practical ethics are also normative. Beauchamp and Childress offer the following remarks on practical ethics: "Often, no straightforward movement from theory or principles to particular judgements is possible. Theory and principles are typically invoked only to help develop action-guides, which are also further shaped by paradigm cases of appropriate behaviour, empirical data, and the like, together with reflection on how to put these influential sources into the most coherent whole" (p. 4).

3. Descriptive ethics: Descriptive ethics investigates moral behaviour and beliefs. It uses standard scientific techniques to study how people reason and act. It studies various beliefs and practices and how they influence our lives. The main goal of descriptive ethics is to describe various moral systems and their influences on behaviour. No judgement is involved, no ordering of things into good and bad, right or wrong. Descriptive ethics are therefore inherently non-normative.

4. Metaethics: Metaethics is the analysis of the language, concepts and methods or reasoning employed in ethics and moral philosophy. It examines meaning of terms such as right, wrong, responsibility, virtue, good, and hope. It also encompasses the study of moral epistemology (the theory of moral knowledge). Metaethics is also non-normative, because its objective is to describe the facts, to establish and verify the *actual condition* in the real world. In comparison, the objective of normative ethics is to establish what the condition in the real world *ought* to be.

*(Note that the use of the word 'normative' is slightly different in ethics than it is in psychology. The 'norm' in psychology is often associated with the average or mean. It is purely descriptive. Normative in ethical terms has to do with establishing a standard of what is to be considered morally correct conduct. It is evaluative rather than descriptive.)

THE MEDICALISATION OF HEALTH

In the last several decades, an increasing number of behaviours which were once considered to belong primarily to the realm of the social sciences are being interpreted in a medical context (Coleman, & Hendry, 1990; Marsh, Rosser, & Harré, 1978). This includes such behaviours as smoking, drinking, and drug abuse, as well as everyday matters such as sleeping habits, eating habits, and ways of communication. Perhaps the broad and widely accepted definition of health adopted by the World Health Organization has contributed to this shift, because it implicates so many types of behaviours. Medicalisation in this context means that medical characteristics are being attributed to an increasing array of behaviours, emotions, and states of being. These behaviours, emotions, and states of being are thus placed in a medical discourse, where they are thought about in a medical context, couched in medical terminology, and considered to be related to medical causes and effects (Broekman, Feldmann, & Van Haute, 1993). The medical discourse is a strong and invasive one, and often precludes or pre-empts thinking about behaviour in other terms once they have been placed in a medical framework. Once within this medical framework, a specific system of expectations and ways of looking at cause and effect are operant. We still expect a great deal from medical technology, and from following the advice of health experts. Although progress in behavioural medicine and other fields is slowly defusing the idea, we often look for specific etiologic explanations for illness or malfunction when manoeuvring within a medical framework. We seem to be seeking the 'magic bullet', based on a one-to-one relationship in which a single cause can be isolated, identified, and dealt with in an appropriate fashion (Laura, & Heaney, 1990). These great expectations tend to foster reliance on a bioreductionist medical model. This model supports the view that scientific technology will eventually offer solutions to most health problems. According to some authors, this reliance on (forthcoming) technological developments impoverishes the individual's autonomous ability to recognise and make sensible use of non-medical health-supporting solutions (Illich, 1975).

In this vein, it is important to recognise that we may not be doing adolescents an unequivocal service by placing a broad array of behaviours within the medical discourse. The question of whether placing behaviours in a medical framework has possible negative or limiting effects on future behavioural repertoire has not, to my knowledge, been addressed empirically. By drawing everyday behaviours into a medical context that allows for health-based interventions, we may be infringing upon privacy, tightening the reins over-zealously, introducing needless complication of simple activities in an already complex world, and contributing to a possibly numbing constriction in perspective. This is certainly not to say that we should call a halt to important interventions for safe sex, healthy diet, and the like. However, as health educators, we continually need to recognise the impact of the unintended consequences of our work, and the prospect that these may overshadow the impact of the intended consequences in the long run.

HEALTH AS A NORM

The shift towards medical explanations inevitably has consequences for intervention techniques and targets. Anti-social behaviours were once combated in social terms, and 'social' or 'normal' behaviour was considered the goal. Now, many of the same behaviours are being combated in medical terms, and 'healthy' behaviour is considered the goal. While the approach may differ, the goals are similar, because healthy behaviour has also come to represent 'normal' and 'social' behaviour. Conversely, unhealthy or risky behaviours are increasingly being experienced as 'anti-social' (Brownell, 1991). So not only is there a progressive medicalisation, but this medicalisation entails a normative and value-laden element.

Health has thus become a normative cultural and social value in Western society (Brownell, 1991). Through the development of antibiotics and improvements in hygiene and living conditions, infectious diseases have been replaced by chronic and degenerative diseases as the prime agents of morbidity and mortality (Laura, & Heaney, 1990). In keeping with this development, disease has come to represent a way of life rather than an epidemic bringing near-certain death (Schepers, & Nievaard, 1990). In this light, sickness and illness have been defined as deviant behaviour (Freidson, 1971), abnormal behaviour, and motivated deviation (Parsons, cited in: Schepers, & Nievaard, 1990). Alongside the medical perspective on health as something to be reinstated if lost or impaired by means of palliative or curative medicine, another perspective on health has taken hold. This perspective has been labelled by some as the social moralist perspective on health (E. van Leeuwen, personal communication). From this perspective, health is something to be actively acquired and retained by means of preventive medicine and healthy behaviours (Brownell, 1991). Prescribed and advised health-related behaviours have become frequent targets for primary prevention interventions, media campaigns, and popular literature. This has extended health-related behaviour beyond the boundaries of treatment compliance in tertiary health care settings. A study done in 1980 showed that 57% of the Dutch population considered health to be the most important thing in life (Schepers, & Nievaard, 1990). Recent statistics from both The Netherlands and the USA show this percentage shooting upwards of 80%. Rising collective health care costs, along with the tenets of personal control and responsibility for health popularised by the wellness movement, have rendered health a personal, social, and public imperative (Brownell, 1991).

Health education, as a by-product of a normative social imperative, teaches a system of values in the process of promoting healthy behaviours and discouraging risky ones. Adolescent health education might thus be construed as a value-laden instrument of socialisation, a tool for the dissemination of norms and values considered important to current society. Directly or inadvertently, in our efforts to improve public health we impart values and moral standards along with our health-related information. We need to know this as health educators, so we can at minimum monitor our output and at maximum understand the differential impact we may have.

THE CONCEPT OF PERSONAL CONTROL AND RESPONSIBILITY

Getting healthy and staying healthy have come to be viewed, to a great extent, as personal responsibilities. Medical science and medical doctors are no longer seen as carrying the sole responsibility for health. As research results exposing numerous links between behaviour and health reach the public, the responsibility to carry out healthy behaviours and avoid risky ones has come to rest with the individual. This places health issues, at least to some extent, firmly outside the doctors' office. This relocation is part of the process referred to as medicalisation. Personal responsibility and control have been shown to be important to health. Declines in death due to heart disease in the USA (Goldman, & Cook, 1984) and suppression of the HIV epidemic in The Netherlands (van Ameijden, van den Hoek, van Haastreacht, & Coutinho, 1994) are examples of improved health which are attributed to life-style change. People who have succeeded in changing their behaviour have been able to improve their health. Even *perceived* control over health-related behaviour has been shown to have a valuable impact on health (Rodin, 1986).

As discussed in Chapter 1, health education for classroom and individual use has been chosen for the research presented in this book. To do intervention on a personal level, we must accept the concept of personal control: personal empowerment will heighten personal control and thus promote personal responsibility for health. The concepts of personal control and responsibility have received resounding empirical backing in the literature (Glanz et al., 1997; Ruwaard, & Kramers, 1993; Tones & Tilford, 1994; Whitehead, 1994). These sources powerfully document the victories of health education and public health strategies to teach behaviour modification and change and to empowering individuals to take personal responsibility for their health. Health education, screening, prevention programmes and so forth have certainly made headway in battles against heart disease, cancer, and a scale of other chronic and infectious illnesses. However, important problems have been identified in relation to the concepts of personal control and responsibility for personal health. I therefore need to temper the above-mentioned acceptation of these concepts with six caveats.

Determining the target

The first caveat is as follows: if we ascribe to the tenet of personal control without reservation, we underestimate social and environmental determinants of health and downplay institutional responsibilities. Health education is easier to implement and more immediately rewarding when carried out on the individual/group level. Danish (1990) remarked that working closely with individuals might make us feel more useful and may make the recipient feel better temporarily. However, if we want to alleviate health risks that are connected to circumstances such as poverty or ignorance, we must eventually intervene in the larger system, or resign ourselves to results that will remain tenuous at best. If we tackle questions of safe sex at the high-school level, but do not ensure access to condoms at the community level, our programme is unlikely to have a lasting effect. If we implement a campaign to improve eating habits in the barrio, but do not ensure the availability of attractive and healthy alternatives, nor the wherewithal to purchase them, our programme is doomed to failure in the long run, no matter how well designed. So, the question becomes, *where* do we intervene? Rappaport (1977, as quoted in Danish, 1990) has defined six levels of the social order. These include the individual, the group, organisations, institutions, communities, and society as a whole. Each level could conceivably be targeted for health intervention. As stated in Danish (1990, p. 96):

> A decision to intervene at one level as opposed to another has implications for the values and goals, conceptual frameworks and strategies of the intervener.

Adherence to the tenet of personal control can and has placed a strong accent upon the individual level of intervention. However, personal responsibility for health cannot take the place of institutional and societal responsibilities. These must go hand in hand.

Feeling better, doing worse

The concept of personal control does not give a complete picture of health determinants. The second caveat I would like to put into place is that the concept of personal control can lead us to overestimate the *extent* of our control over health. This overestimation has been connected to several undesirable outcomes. In Chapter 4, we see that many adolescents are not ready or willing to assume full responsibility for their own health. They are, for the most part, strongly ambivalent on the issue of health-related personal control. Even when adults are willing to assume full responsibility for their health, they do not have full control, for instance, of their gene pool or body type. Overestimation of personal control can induce people to draw inappropriate conclusions, leading to inappropriate choices in personal health care. Moreover, overestimation of personal control over health may lead to hypersensitivity to risk, as well as to the depreciation of social and environmental determinants of health (Brownell, 1991). The concept of personal control encourages the belief that one can control one's health through carrying out a range of healthy behaviours and avoiding a range of risky ones. It has been implicated in the upsurge of a phenomenon referred to by some as 'feeling better and doing worse', and by others as 'worried sick' (Brownell, 1991). As stated in Thomas (1979, p. 38):

> The new danger to our well-being ... is in becoming ... healthy hypochondriacs, living gingerly, worrying ourselves half to death ... back it comes on television or in the weekly newsmagazines, confirming all the fears, instructing us to ... go on a diet. Meditate. Jog. Take two tablets with water. Spring water. If pain persists, if anomie persists, if boredom persists, see your doctor.

A paradox of control

Areas of our lives which once represented personal freedom and individual choices in lifestyle, such as our sex lives, eating habits, sleeping habits, clothing and personal relationships have become medicalised. Many choices are hemmed in by a set of medical and moral imperatives governing the minute details of personal life. However, some of the most salient meanings of behaviour, shown to be powerful predictors of adolescent health-related behaviour (Chapter 5, 8, and 9 of this book) are related to personal freedom, personal choice, and challenging authority. At the time that adolescents are just beginning to gain personal control over many areas of their lives, they are expected to use that control to choose for a presumed healthy lifestyle, the elements of which are dictated only to a certain extent by biomedical research. This presents a paradoxical situation, a contradiction in terms, and illustrates my third caveat on the tenet of personal control. Freedom from parental control is thus not followed by freedom of personal choice, but by a limited freedom to restrict oneself to a particular set of choices which society not only advises, but also *expects* the adolescent to internalise. For adolescents, this paradox can be experienced as frustrating and unfair. Resistance to these restrictions may lead adolescents to imbue precisely those behaviours which health education seeks to avoid with salient meanings, disengaging them from any health implications and giving them a great deal of allure.

Personal control and social justice

The fourth caveat is that acceptance of the tenet of personal control needs to be accompanied by acceptance of reciprocal responsibility. The relationship of personal responsibility to social and environmental influences raises the issue of rights versus reciprocal responsibilities or duties, which is embedded in the concept of social justice. Several interpretations of the concept of social justice have been offered by various philosophers (Beauchamp, & Childress, 1989; Elster, 1989). One of the interpretations most cited in the context of health education is Rawls' concept of social justice, which is based on a particular perspective on equal opportunity and on the idea of 'rights reciprocated by responsibility' (Beauchamp, & Childress, 1989; Laura, & Heaney, 1990). According to Rawls, health status cannot be controlled by a given social order, but the level of health will be affected by the provision, or lack of provision regarding health and health care within that social order. Health will thus continue to be influenced by the immediate environment and the surrounding society (Green, & Kreuter, 1991). Therefore, to optimally take responsibility for one's health implies sharing responsibility for the societal structure and the environment. If one accepts the concept of personal responsibility and the influence of society and environment upon health, one must also accept that the individual bears a responsibility towards the community. Reciprocally, the community bears a responsibility to ensure that individuals are in the position to exercise autonomy, in other words to make educationally informed decisions about issues relating to their health. If the responsibility for health is thus conceptualised as one shared between individual and society, health education becomes essential to ensure that each individual is prepared to contribute not only to the maintenance of personal health, but to the dialogue which will shape health policies.

Blaming the victim

The fifth caveat on the tenet of personal control is its implication in a growing tendency referred to as 'Blaming the victim'. 'Blaming the victim' occurs when adherence to the principle of personal control leads to blaming people for their own illnesses and physical or psychological problems (Brownell, 1991; Laura, & Heaney, 1990). As Colman states (quoted in Laura, & Heaney, 1990, p.171):

> Positive health is not something that one human can hand to or require of another. Positive health can be achieved only through intelligent effort. Absent that effort, health professionals can only insulate the individual from more catastrophic results of his ignorance, self-indulgence, or lack of motivation.

This new health mentality bears moral overtones: Those who are healthy and those who engage in the right behaviours are good. Those who are ill or do not engage in the right behaviours have let down their families, their society, themselves, and are assumed to have personal weaknesses (Brownell, 1991). In this view, if health is not achieved and retained, it is at least to a certain extent a question of personal blame. If people lead a healthy lifestyle, eat the right food, and maintain a proper ratio between exercise, rest, work, and reproduction, they will be healthy. If they do not and are not healthy, it is their own fault.

The attribution of responsibility to the victim has been shown to incur behavioural consequences. When adolescents believe that someone is personally responsible for his or her own adversity, they tend to react with anger rather than with sympathy. These visceral reactions have been shown to influence behaviour. A chain reaction occurs, beginning with attribution of blame. If attribution of blame or responsibility falls upon the victim, anger ensues and the adolescent will generally refuse to offer help. If the victim is not perceived to be responsible for adversity, sympathy ensues and adolescents are willing to help (Caprara, Pastorelli, & Weiner, 1997; Weiner, 1995). By allocating responsibility to the victim, adolescents divest themselves of any responsibility for that person. Thinking through the implications of these findings, we see how victim blaming can lead to a decline in social justice as defined by Rawls.

The evolution of victim blaming has been ascribed to the rising collective costs of medical treatment and to the notion of reciprocal rights (Crawford, 1977). Personal irresponsibility in health-related behaviours is seen by many as anti-social because it raises health costs for the entire community and has a negative influence on the just distribution of relatively scarce commodities. An emphasis on changing individual factors to the exclusion of systemic factors can lead to absolving management from responsibility for work conditions and job demands. It can lead us to absolve the government from responsibility to support social programmes and research into the social causes of ill health. It can deceive us into overlooking opportunities to deal with significant environmental determinants of disease (Brownell, 1991).

If the content of health education is limited to information on individual behaviour modification, it may contribute to an exclusive focus on personal control. During adolescence, cognitive abilities to understand difficult principles related to health develop together with the moral framework within which health and health-related behaviours will be understood (Cobb, 1992; Gilligan, 1988; Kohlberg, 1984). In this light, the role of health education is once again extended beyond dissemination of purely health-related information. Health education entails normative and moralistic messages. In adolescent health education, these messages are transmitted to an impressionable group at a formative interval in their lives. In this way, the tasks involved in adolescent health education tend to expand. Making an informed contribution to moral development becomes part and parcel of the endeavour. Preparing adolescents for gradual assumption of a realistic measure of personal responsibility remains one of the central tasks. As we have seen, this involves the examination of issues relating to social justice in order to contribute to a fundamental understanding of the balance between health-related rights and responsibilities.

Personal responsibility for health and minority status

One last caveat must be placed concerning the influence of the concept of personal control upon issues of social justice and victim blaming. Research in developed countries has repeatedly shown that the health of minority adolescents is generally poorer than the health of their dominant-culture peers (Mackenbach, 1992; Netherlands Central Bureau of Statistics, 1992; Wilson et al., 1997b). The jury is still out on the nature of the relationship between these persistent differences and ethnicity, culture, and socio-economic status. It is clear that these differences cannot be attributed solely to (lack of) personal control or (refusal to take) personal responsibility of personal health. Different relationships between biology, culture, behaviour, and health are showing up for different cultural groups (Wilson et al., 1997b). As is documented in Chapter 4, the study of health behaviours and the creation of effective lesson materials cannot be undertaken for different ethnic groups simultaneously, unless the knowledge and funding are in place to consider the needs of each target group separately and thoroughly.

CHARACTERISTICS OF INFORMATION ON HEALTH: WHICH BEHAVIOURS ARE HEALTHY?

At the core of the ethical issues surrounding health education are the characteristics of the information upon which it must be based. This information is sometimes comprehensible, sometimes controversial, and sometimes stable, which complicates the development of dependable health education programmes for all but the most straightforward behaviours. For instance, smoking is not healthy. This has been proven beyond reasonable doubt. However, drawing conclusions from the available information on other, more complex networks of behaviour, poses elaborate problems.

Sometimes comprehensible: Different disciplines, different jargons

Those who want to utilise the newest research on health-related behaviour may be confronted with information that is difficult to access and difficult to comprehend. The people responsible for health education are usually not researchers in relevant health fields, such as human nutrition, biochemistry, or medical biology. Sometimes necessary information is inaccessible to the uninitiated in the field because they just do not know where to look for it. If health educators can access the information they need, there are still problems of comprehensibility. Health educators are not necessarily familiar with the various paradigms or versed in the particular scientific jargon of the myriad of scientific fields they need to tap for their work. The information they need to use is often detailed, and in trying to popularise it or make it comprehensible to the general public, information often gets taken out of context.

It often loses meaningful and necessary elements in the translation, without which the information becomes less useful, less clear, or just plain wrong.

Sometimes controversial: Lack of consensus on health-related information

Controversies about which behaviours should be considered healthy or risky have been receiving more attention in the media, in scientific journals, in textbooks. For instance, the jury is still out concerning the amount of sugars or fats (and the kind of fats) that can be considered acceptable/optimal in our diets. The controversy still rages on the safety of various sugar substitutes. The usefulness of vitamin C and other supplements to our diet has yet to be agreed upon (Hamilton, Whitney, & Sizer, 1991). For the health educator, this lack of consensus makes it difficult to reach well-founded decisions concerning the precise behaviours to be promoted or prevented. Professional training in health education may not provide the expertise to make independent choices between, for instance, the various amounts, strategies and forms of calcium intake which best aid in the prevention of osteoporosis. Because of lack of consensus in the relevant fields, gathering information is not simply a question of looking it up in an appropriate source. It may require extensive literature study, and inevitably making choices that health educators may not be equipped to make. This points to the imperative of multidisciplinary teams for the construction of health education interventions. However, even multidisciplinary teams can be deadlocked by controversial subject matter. To aid in the construction of the lesson materials used in this research, 14 experts (5 doctors, 6 nutritionists, and 3 dieticians) filled in an open questionnaire on nutrition. On basic issues such as whether or not sugar intake should be limited, whether or not processed drinks or drinks with unnecessary additives should be avoided, and whether or not moderate alcohol consumption should be discouraged for adolescents between 12 and 16 years of age, the scores were fairly evenly distributed between 'agree', 'not sure', and 'disagree'. There was no particular relationship evident between the various answer categories and different educational backgrounds.

Sometimes stable: Mutability of health-related information

The perpetual barrage of new findings on health-related behaviour causes constant changes in the list of behaviours which are considered healthy, and also the interrelationships between various behaviours and health. A case in point is the discovery that consumption of partially hydrogenated fats, long advocated for their cholesterol-lowering ability, is linked to undesirable side effects and may even increase blood cholesterol levels (Blonz, 1993). For health educators, these frequent changes pose severe obstacles to staying well informed, keeping the public well informed, and keeping health education materials up to date. The use of obsolete materials or interventions based on less than current information can lead to the development of beliefs, opinions, and behaviours that will require rectification, involving the complications and difficulties inherent in changing them (Chapter 3).

THE ISSUE OF VOLUNTARINESS

We assume, despite the many caveats mentioned here, that health education is one of the basic requirements for the adequate provision of health services, and that it provides an essential tool for improving public health. If we go with this assumption, and commit to undertake health education interventions, we want our interventions to be effective. As discussed in Chapter 1, the definition of an effective health education intervention is one that leads to voluntary behaviour modification. Green, Kreuter, Deeds, and Partridge (quoted in McKenzie, & Lurs, 1993, p. 3) define health education as "any combination of learning experiences designed to facilitate voluntary adaptations of behaviour conducive to health". This element of voluntariness is echoed by the Joint Committee on Health Education Terminology (1990, p. 103), which defines health education as enabling people to "... voluntarily make decisions, modify behaviours, and change social conditions in ways which are health enhancing". Voluntariness touches on the issue of respect for autonomy. The principle of respect for autonomy obligates professionals to disclose information and to promote understanding and voluntariness. Autonomous actions should not be subjected to controlling constraints by others (Beauchamp, & Childress, 1989). McKenzie, and Lurs (1993) delineate what they have called a 'hierarchy of autonomy' in their book on health promotion (Table 2.1).

Moving from 'A' to 'D' implies a diminishing 'amount' of autonomy. In school-based health education, the target group (students) is not usually involved in setting objectives. Teachers and parents are not necessarily consulted. Objectives are often set by an umbrella organisation or institution, such as the CDC or the NIH or are a function of the lesson materials employed. This precludes category 'A' interventions according to Table 2.1. If we consider the overview offered in Chapter 3 of theories and models of behaviour change often employed in health education, several of them could be located at 'B', most at 'C', and a few, such as those that advocate the use of fear messages, might even

TABLE 2.1

Hierarchy of autonomy

A. Facilitation (assisting in achieving objectives set by a target group)
B. Persuasion (argue and reason)
C. Manipulation (modify the environment around a person or the psychic disposition of the person
D. Coercion (threat of deprivation)

(Adapted from McKenzie, & Lurs, 1993, p.186)

be considered to be located at 'D'. These and other theories of behavioural change do not focus primarily on the facilitation of choice. Rather, their focus is on the manipulation of attitudes, beliefs, perceptions, motivations, or meanings in order to initiate behavioural change. These types of manipulations are seldom made explicit to the target group, and not always explained to the teachers who implement the programmes. Theory functions in the background: it is implicit. The Society for Public Health Education (SOPHE) (1976) has drawn up a code of ethics, in which it stands that: "I will support change by choice, not by coercion". However, it can be questioned whether the use of an intervention based on any of the prevalent theories of behaviour change is in compliance with this code.

DISCUSSION

Health education may contribute to an overly medicalised and constricting view of behaviour, may have a value-laden and normative function, may contribute to an unrealistic estimation of the extent and effectiveness of personal control, and may infringe upon autonomy. Under these conditions, perhaps we must question whether we have the right to attempt to change behaviour on the basis of impermanent and incomplete information. At the same time, we must question whether we have the right not to. Health education has made a substantial contribution to the welfare of others. It has aided in the accomplishment of behavioural change in several areas, and this behavioural change has improved health (Brownell, 1991). The principle of beneficence from the field of ethics refers to a moral obligation to act for the benefit of others or an obligation to help others further their welfare. The principle of non-malificence refers to a moral obligation to refrain from doing harm (Beauchamp, & Childress, 1989). In health education, as in medical practice, these two principles may be at odds, and it becomes a question of balancing the projected benefits and drawbacks of a planned intervention and taking periodic inventory as the project proceeds. The ethical question that must repeatedly be asked is: "Do the ends justify the means?"

It is not unusual for health educators to be faced with decisions about ethics when designing programmes, and therefore it is important for them to be aware of issues such as those discussed here (McKenzie, & Lurs, 1993). The recipients of health education are directly affected by these issues, and it might serve health education well to address this. One approach is to include open discussion of these issues as part of the process of health education. While there are no simple ways to settle these issues, much can be done within the context of lesson materials. We can educate people concerning the changeable nature of health-related information, the pros and cons of the concept of personal control and responsibility, the normative aspects of health education. We can open up the discussion on the pitfalls of medicalisation, and on issues surrounding voluntariness. Health education that approaches these issues openly and encourages critical, evaluative thought offers recipients a firm base from which a broad behavioural repertoire can be built and from which well-informed, autonomous decisions on health-related matters can be made.

CHAPTER THREE

Theories and models used in adolescent health research and education

INTRODUCTION

The practical value of theory in health education is immense. The use of theories helps to build a broad base of understanding, adds coherence and effectiveness to our endeavours, and aids in the process of evaluation (Glanz, Lewis, & Rimer, 1990; Glanz et al., 1997; Green, & Kreuter, 1991). With this conviction, it is essential to review extant theories used in the study of health-related behaviour in order to ground the ensuing research and interventions firmly in theory. At present, however, a gap exists between theoretical and applied science in health behaviour research and education (Glanz et al., 1990, 1997; Hochbaum, Sorenson, & Loring, 1992; Jessor, 1993). Narrowing this gap is undoubtedly thwarted by the hyperabundance of available theories and models. For example, Cummings, Becker, and Maille (1980) distilled six factors from 14 models of health behaviour involving 104 constructs. In 1990, Glanz et al. reviewed 116 theory-based articles published between 1986 and 1988 in two of the leading journals in health education, and found 51 distinct theoretical formulations. Fishbein and his colleagues tried to cut across the plethora of available theories and identify a set of key variables that accounted for most variance in health behaviour research. They set out a group of eight key variables: intention, ability/skill, norms, environmental constraints, anticipated outcomes, self-standards, emotion, and self-efficacy (Glanz et al., 1997). More recently, Glanz and her colleagues reviewed articles from relevant journals published between 1992 and 1994. This time they identified 66 different models. Twenty-one of these were mentioned eight or more times in the reviewed literature (Glanz et al., 1997).

In spite of this awesome pluriformity, theory-based research is fundamental to the progress of understanding in the field. A good theory provides a conceptual

Box 3.1: Theories and models

What is a theory? Theory has been defined in various ways throughout the history of the philosophy of science. Here is a simple definition of *theory*:

(1) "A theory is a unified explanation for discrete observations that might otherwise be viewed as unrelated or contradictory" (Patten, 1997, p. 27).

In this conception, deduction is a part of theory forming and use (first form a theory, then deduce hypotheses from the theory, then test them), as is induction (first observe events, then develop a theory that seems to fit them). It doesn't offer any information on ideas of cause and effect, testability, or other demands of rigorous science.

A more comprehensive definition of *theory* is:

(2) "...a system of logically coherent, explicitly not conflicting, statements, interpretations and concepts concerning a selected aspect of reality, that are formulated so that it is possible to derive testable hypotheses from them" (de Groot, 1961, p. 42, my translation).

In his book, de Groot emphasises the importance of testable hypotheses. He views both induction and deduction as part of the theory-forming process. Note the importance of systematic inquiry. In his view, theory can facilitate logical and systematic coherence of research in any area. He sees theory as both a tool and an objective.

Here is very demanding definition of *theory*:

(3) "...a fairly comprehensive, causal explanation"
(Viera, Pollock, & Golez, 1998, p.16).

You are beginning to see that any definition of *theory* you get will be influenced by characteristics of the 'definer'. Your 'definer's' field of expertise will affect the definition of theory you get, and the field of expertise is often tied to differing opinions on the nature of cause and effect. Definitions from the physical and biological sciences tend to veer away from description and expect a theory to lead to laws (that will always hold) and directional explanations of cause and effect (the "A leads inexorably to B" kind of cause and effect). This is tied into the positivist opinions that the nature of causes can be truly grasped. Social scientists might also refer to cause and effect, but modify their conception to refer to 'relationships between phenomena'. The directionality is less emphatic, A does not always lead to B, but there might be a relationship. This difference in conceptualisation of cause and effect is due to the nature of the phenomena under study in social scientist. Phenomena in the social-scientific world do not lend themselves to single cause explanations or explanations that always hold true. Social scientists "are willing to assert that causes have a real nature, albeit one that can only be imperfectly grasped" (Cook, & Campbell, 1979, p. 30). Cook and Campbell offer a lengthy and interesting introduction on how the scientific-philosophical school which informed your training or education (or to which you subscribe) will influence how you understand the concepts of cause and effect.

Glanz and her colleagues (1997, paraphrased from p. 21–22) define *theory* as follows:

(4) A theory is a set of interrelated concepts, definitions, and propositions that presents a systematic view of events or situations by specifying relations among constructs in order to explain and predict the events or situations.

In this conception of theory, the idea of generalisability, or broad application, is important, as is the idea of testability. Prediction finally pops up explicitly here—albeit in the social-scientific sense of the word. Here we are not referring to perfect one-on-one predictions or constant unidirectional relationships, but rather to a percentage of explained variance, to relationships that explain behaviour better than chance. We are predicting some of the behaviour for some of the people some of the time. A *theory* defined in this way will describe at least and predict at best. This last definition is the one adhered to in this book.

A model is a formalised theory. It postulates which constructs one needs from a theory in order to make deductions or predictions about a selected aspect of reality. A model also specifies the nature of the relationships between the constructs (de Groot, 1961). You can usually draw a model using circles (for the constructs) and arrows (to specify the relationships). Not all theories lend themselves directly to making models.

framework to examine the interrelationship between constructs (Brown et al., 1991; Glanz et al., 1990, 1997). A good theory facilitates the estimation of the relative impact of the various constructs, which in turn can guide further intervention and research (Bentler, & Speckart, 1979; Brown et al., 1991; de Groot, 1961). In adolescent health research and education, a good theory can guide development of interventions by delineating factors and determinants to be studied, by identifying facilitating situations and relevant processes, by guiding timing and sequencing, and by indicating possible methods of intervention and evaluation (Glanz et al., 1990, 1997).

The question is: Which theories are 'good' theories for adolescent populations? Although there are many approaches imaginable to this question, let me propose the following six criteria for a 'good' theory in adolescent health behaviour and education research (Spruijt-Metz, 1998b). According to these six criteria, a good theory is one that (1) consistently describes, explains, and predicts behaviour well, (2) has prescriptive potential for behavioural influence and change, (3) is relevant for the target group, (4) is empirically testable, (5) is parsimonious, and (6) is user-friendly. Let's look at these criteria more closely.

The first one, involving description and prediction, is related to McGuire's (1983) concept of ecological validity. A descriptive theory is one that conforms to reality when you test it. It tells you something about the behaviour you have studied. A predictive theory yields constructs that not only describe behaviour, but can also be used to predict it in the future. This is essential to be able to develop effective interventions that use present findings to influence future behaviour.

The second criterion concerns the prescriptive content of a theory. A prescriptive theory tells you which constructs can be changed, how to go about changing them, and how these changes will in turn affect the targeted behaviours. There are many great theories of behaviour that implicate constructs (such as socio-economic status and gender) which cannot be directly influenced by health education efforts. These theories are invaluable in the quest for greater knowledge and useful in the larger context of health promotion. However, to design and implement health education, theories identifying constructs that can be manipulated and changed by health education are needed.

The third criterion, that of applicability to the target group, is often overlooked in adolescent health education. A theory may predict certain health-related behaviours with great success in adults, but may not do so for adolescents. A theory may have been developed using samples of Caucasian American college students and predict their behaviour adequately. This same theory might fail miserably or need considerable adjustment for use with younger adolescents or for different socio-economic or ethnic groups (Pasnick, 1997).

The fourth and fifth criteria are related. Testability implies that the constructs involved are measurable. This means that the constructs of the chosen theory can be operationalised successfully and measured responsibly (Cook, & Campbell, 1979; Cook, Anson, & Walchli, 1993). The concept of testability (or falsifiability or refutability) emanates from Sir Karl Popper's work (Popper, 1976). For a theory to be testable, it must be possible to refute it using empirical evidence. So 'It will rain or not rain here tomorrow' is not testable simply because it cannot be refuted; whereas the statement, 'It will rain here tomorrow' is testable (Popper, 1959, p. 41). Popper's ideas on testability stemmed in part from a growing dissatisfaction with many of the prevailing psychological theories. These theories included so many variables and were couched in such vague language that almost any evidence could be construed to represent 'verification'. They were not 'demarcated'—there was no true boundary between empirical scientific thought and metaphysics (or, as Popper put it, between scientific theories and pseudo-scientific theories). Here is the link between criteria 4 and 5. A testable theory in this sense cannot involve too many constructs. It must thus be parsimonious. In de Groot's opinion, as in Popper's, the concept of parsimony (or the principle of economy) is central to the development of a 'good' theory. According to both of these distinguished thinkers, a theory should strive to be as simple as possible. A theory should explain and predict a particular (well-demarcated) phenomenon with as few constructs and assumptions as possible (de Groot, 1961, p. 73). Finally, a parsimonious theory has a better chance of conforming to the last of the six criteria.

The last criterion demands that a theory be user-friendly. A user-friendly theory is useable and useful in the field. It can be implemented in health education, practitioners can follow the logic, it is plausible and internally consistent (Glanz et al., 1997).

While a great deal of valuable research is being done in the area of adolescent health, fully developed formal theories have not yet been attained in the field. The usefulness of any particular theory therefore depends on the particular behaviour to be studied and the circumstances under which it is being studied (Glanz et al.,

1990). At best, the present social scientific theories on health-related behaviour identify the determinants governing the phenomena of interest (Bandura, 1986). McGuire (1983) has suggested that research at this stage in the development of the field should attempt to delineate the contexts, or conditions, under which hypotheses hold, rather than to aspire to the logical positivist ideal of formulating right or wrong hypotheses in any absolute sense. From the contextualist perspective, we are looking for an understanding of what works best under which conditions. The subject matter remains too complex and changeable, and the effectiveness of existing programmes too sporadic, to warrant exclusive replication of well-researched programmes or bias towards one (or several) extant theories (Glanz et al., 1990). Choosing a 'good' theory in this perspective depends upon the settings, subjects, and behaviour of interest on one hand, and upon the limits of the available theories on the other.

The current theories employed in adolescent health research have divergent strong points, as will be demonstrated in the course of this review. Frequently voiced criticisms of these theories are that they often assume a basically rational person and a (chrono)logical, chain-of-events model of behaviour (Spruijt-Metz, 1995; Stacy, Bentler, & Flay, 1994). This basically rational person is one who is assumed to make reasonable choices in an autonomous fashion according to available information (Beauchamp, & Childress, 1989). The chain-of-events model of behaviour places the rational person in a rational world, where logical, linear, relationships between knowledge, cognitions, motivations, beliefs, attitudes and intentions lead to behaviour. It is doubtful that these assumptions hold consistently for adolescent populations (Kirscht, 1983). Several researchers have suggested that less rational, more emotional determinants of behaviour which encompass the adolescent's perception of the world and its guiding mechanisms, need to be addressed in adolescent health research (Brown et al., 1991; Hølund, 1990b; Perry, & Kelder, 1992). These remarks will function as a *Leitmotiv* in the ensuing theoretical review.

CHOOSING THEORIES

A complete overview of all available theories on health education and research is beyond the scope of this or any other book (Glanz et al., 1997). Therefore, a selection of prominent theories has been made according to their influence, relevance, and usefulness in adolescent health education and research. Selecting theories and models entailed a number of difficult decisions. For the most part, only theories that have been used in recent (after 1988) empirical research within an adolescent population have been included. The few exceptions to this criterion reflect a purely subjective choice of theories that the present author considers essential to the field. Another criterion for inclusion was that the theory be suited specifically to the limited area of health education, as opposed to theories designed for the broader area of health promotion, which subsumes the field of health education (McKenzie, & Lurs, 1993). Leading theoretical frameworks in health promotion, such as the PRECEDE PROCEED model (Green, & Kreuter, 1991), and the Health Action model (Tones, & Tilford, 1994), have therefore been excluded. Resilience theories have contributed profoundly to recent research on adolescent health. For instance, the National Longitudinal Study of Adolescent Health (Add Health) is informed to a great extent by these theories (Blum, & Rinehart, 1997; Haggerty, Sherrod, Garmezy, & Rutter, 1996; Resnick et al., 1997). The breadth of the endeavour required to design intervention programmes based on the resilience paradigm reaches beyond the realm of health education and deep into health promotion paradigms. Therefore, the network of resilience theories has been excluded from this review. Further choices were made on the basis of the heuristic proposed by Glanz et al. (1990, 1997), who categorise theories according to important units of health education practice: the individual, the interpersonal or group level, and the community or aggregate level. Because the research presented here is concerned with health education at the individual level using more or less conventional lesson materials, theories and models at the individual level receive the most attention. Only one interpersonal theory, the Social–Cognitive theory, is included, because of widespread use of some of its constructs in individual level intervention. Community level theories are considered part of health promotion and are not included.

The theories discussed here are ordered into five groups: social–cognitive approaches, belief-based approaches, attitude-based approaches, theories designed specifically to explain adolescent behaviour, and theories offering general frameworks for multi-theoretical approaches. Several of the theories appear as models, in which substantive theories are translated into specified constructs and their interrelations (Bentler, 1978). For each theory or model discussed, the following four steps will be followed: (1) presentation of the basic theory, (2) description of developments and additions, (3) review of recent research results in adolescent health research and education, and (4) discussion of relevant criticism. In the review of research and the discussion of criticism, attention will be accorded to both theoretical and methodological issues.

Box 3.2: From constructs through operationalisation to variables

It is important to distinguish systematically between constructs and variables. A theory always identifies constructs, and *never* identifies variables. Constructs are the rich, theoretical and abstract concepts yielded by any social scientific theory (Kidder, & Judd, 1986). Constructs are ideas, like 'self efficacy' in the first theory to be discussed below. Constructs in social science cannot usually be held in your hand or pointed out directly in reality. Therefore, they often cannot be measured directly. However, in order to use constructs in research, we need to be able to measure them. To do this, scientists devise concrete representations that are, of necessity, approximations of what is meant by the construct. How a particular scientist represents a construct in his or her research will always be influenced by how that particular scientist understands or interprets the theory, field of interest, knowledge base, funding limitations, etc. Any one construct can be measured in countless different ways, because any abstract idea can be represented in countless different ways. Each of these representations will refer to the same *construct*, but will produce a different *variable*. Many different representations of the same construct will hold some degree of truth or validity, and usually none of them will be entirely satisfying.

The process of moving from abstract construct to concrete variable is called 'operationalisation'. Variables are thus referred to as 'operationalisations' or 'operational definitions' of constructs. When we study a construct such as 'power', we must operationalise the construct in some way. We may use a questionnaire, interview, observation, or any other research technique in order to contrive our variable from the original construct. These different measurement techniques all have their specific influences on the validity of our measurements, or the accuracy of our observations (Cook, & Campbell, 1979). Furthermore, we may choose to represent 'power' in many different ways, depending on our research questions and our understanding of the construct. 'Power' might be conceptualised as the amount of influence one has at home, or at work, or in the neighbourhood, or in the media, or in politics (Kidder, & Judd, 1986). There is no way we can cover the whole spectrum of possible operationalisations of 'power' in our research, nor will they all be relevant to our particular bit of research. Our contrived variable will form but one of many possible representations of the construct 'power'. Since any single construct has multiple possible variables, we must always consider our variables to be partial representations of the constructs upon which they are based.

Variables often have the same name as the construct they are meant to represent, which makes things very confusing. Because there are countless different ways to operationalise any social scientific construct, the literature is full of profoundly divergent variables with the same name (because they derive from the same construct). Often the actual variables will be 'invisible', at least to some extent, unless the questionnaires are printed in full. We are frequently left knowing the construct that the research refers to, but guessing at the variable that was actually measured.

It is essential to keep this in mind while reading this review of research: The same construct can and will be operationalised in different ways by different researchers, yielding different variables. These variables might all have the same name because they represent the same construct, but they will have very different measurement characteristics, exhibit inconsistent levels of validity, and they will often represent different aspects or conceptualisations of the same construct. Needless to say, how (well) a construct is operationalised or measured influences its usefulness in research and in predicting behaviour.

SOCIAL–COGNITIVE APPROACHES

The Social–Cognitive theory

The Social Learning theory, predecessor of the Social–Cognitive theory (SCT), was first introduced by Miller and Dollard in 1941. The theory was based on the mechanistic, 'black box' behaviourist approach to learning and behaviour proposed by Hull, and modified by Skinner (Perry, Baranowski, & Parcel, 1990). In these theoretical approaches, behaviours are referred to as operants. Operants operate on the environment, bringing about either reinforcements (rewards) or punishments, which in turn either increase or decrease the likelihood of occurrence of the operant behaviour. According to the stimulus-response hypothesis formulated by Skinner, the frequency of behaviour is determined by its consequences (or reinforcements). No mentalistic concepts such as 'reasoning' or 'thinking' are needed to explain behaviour. Two streams of health-related research emanated from Miller and Dollard's original theory. One is Rotter's Social Learning theory (Rotter, 1966), in which the locus of control construct was developed. Another is Bandura's Social Learning theory, renamed the Social–Cognitive theory (SCT) in 1986, in which the concept of self-efficacy was developed.

In 1977, Bandura published his refutation of the adequacy of traditional learning theory principles for understanding learning, and reconceptualised human learning and motivation in terms of cognitive processes (Bandura, 1977a, 1977b). In doing so, Bandura shifted the focus of his Social Learning theory away from the stimulus-response theories and towards the more cognitive theories. Cognitive theories emphasise subjective expectations, and are generally termed 'value-expectancy' theories. Most of the theories discussed here are value-expectancy theories, as are most of the prevalent theories in current health behaviour research. In value-expectancy theories, behaviour is considered to be a function of the subjective value of an outcome and the subjective expectation (or probability) that a particular behaviour will achieve that outcome. The crucial assumption is that outcome expectancies influence behaviour. Several methodological and conceptual questions have been raised regarding the measurement and function of expectancies, the ramifications of simultaneously examining the predictive power of different specific expectancies and more general expectancies, the differential impact of negative and positive expectancies, and the actual position of expectancies in the various models in relation to behaviour (Stacy, MacKinnin, & Pentz, 1993). Perhaps the most serious problem which has been documented is the difficulty of evaluating the direct causation of behaviour by expectancies (Stacy, Newcomb, & Bentler, 1991). Nevertheless, the value-expectancy approach has yielded valuable, interesting, and abundant research in the field of health behaviour and health education.

According to Bandura, behaviour is determined by incentives and expectancies. Incentives, consequences, or reinforcements (the terms are often used interchangeably) are defined as the subjective value placed upon a particular object or outcome. Behaviour is governed by the subjective interpretation of its consequences. A distinction has been made between three types of expectancies: environmental, outcome, and self-efficacy expectancies (Bandura, 1986; Rosenstock, Strecher, & Becker, 1988). Environmental expectancies are beliefs about how events are connected, about cause and effect. An outcome expectancy is a person's estimate that a given behaviour will lead to certain outcomes. An efficacy expectancy, or perceived self-efficacy, pertains to convictions about one's personal competence to successfully perform the behaviour required to produce desired outcomes. Self-efficacy does not reflect a person's actual skills, but a person's judgement of what one can do with whatever skills one possesses. It relates to beliefs about capabilities to perform specific behaviours in particular situations, and does not refer to a general trait. Self-efficacy can vary on three dimensions: magnitude (according to the difficulty of the task), generality (according to the generalisation of efficacy expectations to other domains of behaviour), and strength (according to how certain one is about one's ability to perform a given task). Figure 3.1 offers definitions of some of the SCT-specific terminology, and shows the relationship between the person, behaviour, outcome, and expectations as conceptualised by Bandura.

In terms of health behaviour, people will change their behaviour if they believe that present behaviour poses a threat to a valued outcome (environmental expectancy), that the new behaviour will lead to the desired outcome (outcome expectancy), and that they are capable of carrying out the new behaviour (self-efficacy expectancy).

Most of the theories discussed in this review have added constructs over the years as the theories develop, or borrowed constructs from other theories, most frequently from the SCT. Self-efficacy is the central construct in the SCT. Self-efficacy is often employed in health research independently of the rest of the theory, or in conjunction with other theories, such as the Health Belief model (Kelly, Zyzanske, & Almegano, 1991), the theory of Reasoned Action (Kok, de Vries, Mudde, & Strecher, 1991), and the Protection Motivation theory (Maddux, & Rogers, 1983). According to Bandura, efficacy expectations influence cognitive, motivational, affective and selectional processes (Bandura, 1992). Self-efficacy is particularly attractive to health researchers and educators because of this assumed broad influence upon behaviour, because measurement of perceived self-efficacy is easier than measurement of actual skills, and because self-efficacy is eminently manipulable (Froman, & Owen, 1991). Efficacy expectations can be learned from four sources: (a) actual success at the task (performance accomplishments), (b) vicarious learning, (c) verbal persuasion, and (d) interpretation of physiological cues (Becker, 1990). All four of these sources are alterable, and to some extent accessible to classroom teachers. The SCT is often considered a practical and useful addition to health research because it offers this prescriptive specificity on how to change behaviour, which is uncommon in many of the theories that may explain or predict behaviour more elegantly.

Discussion of research results in health behaviour research requires a prefacing word concerning the difference between intentions to behave and actual behaviour. Intentions to behave are often measured along with or instead of actual behaviour, and represent subjective evaluations of future behavioural plans. Intentions are usually easier to measure and predict than behaviour. Needless to say, people do not always carry out their intentions, and the empirical relationship between

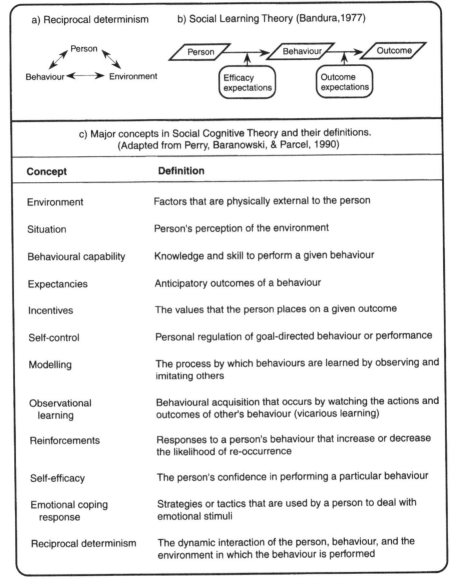

FIG. 3.1   Social Cognitive theory (SCT) (formerly Social Learning theory).
(Adapted from Bandura, 1977b, 1986).

intentions and behaviour has proven to be an inconsistent one (Eagly, & Chaiken, 1993). In several studies, intentions have performed moderately to poorly as predictors of behaviour (Godin, & Shepard, 1990; Hoogstraten, de Haan, & ter Horst, 1985). While van den Putte (1993) claims that this lack of correspondence between intentions and behaviour is mainly a measurement problem related to the fact that intentions change between measurement and behaviour, he admits that there is no easy solution to the problem. Be it due to practical measurement problems or theoretical weakness, intentions are generally mediocre predictors of actual behaviour. A theory may predict intentions without being able to predict behaviour.

In general, the predictive power of self-efficacy in adolescent health research is modest, but consistent, although there are no standardised measurements of self-efficacy. The studies reported here usually employed several Likert-type questions on various dimensions of self-efficacy, such as magnitude and strength, which were gleaned from Bandura's theory. In a study of the effects of the Child and Adolescent Trial for Cardiovascular Health (CATCH) on physical activity, self-efficacy showed only sporadic relations to any changes in physical activity (Edmundson, Parcel, Feldman, & Elder, 1996). De Vries, Dijkstra, and Kuhlman (1988) studied the unique contributions of attitude, social norms and self-efficacy to the prediction of smoking behaviours in a sample of Dutch adolescents. They found that self-efficacy explained 9% of the variance in behaviour, although smokers and non-smokers did not differ in efficacy expectations over all situations. In a predominantly adolescent Dutch population, den Hertog (1992) reports that self-efficacy explained less than 1% of the variance in intentions to carry out various injury preventive behaviours during sport practice. Previous behaviour explained more variance in behavioural intentions than self-efficacy, attitudes, beliefs, norms, outcome expectancies, risk perception, anxiety for injuries, locus of control or sensation seeking. Basen-Engquist and Parcel (1992) found that self-efficacy accounted for 5% of the variance in frequency of condom use in a survey of Texas ninth graders. Other studies of health-related behaviour in adolescent populations show more or less similar results. Self-efficacy rarely predicts a great deal of variance in behaviour. However, it usually offers a significant unique contribution to the prediction.

The SCT has been described as Eurocentric, and its usefulness for interventions with minority youth and lower SES populations has been recently questioned (Resnicow, Braithwaite, & Kuo, 1997; Resnicow, Robinson, & Frank, 1996). Approaches based on the SCT were found to be largely ineffective in changing behaviour through modifying self-efficacy in minority youth populations. However, Resnicow and his colleagues maintain that the SCT could potentially be adapted for the development of culturally sensitive interventions. In their review of the literature, Wilson et al. (1997b) found mixed results of dietary interventions for minority adolescents aimed at improving self-efficacy. Some interventions improved self-efficacy, but this did not consistently lead to changes in dietary behaviour.

While the SCT is regularly a focus of lively philosophical discussions (Bandura, 1990, 1992), it is not a regular recipient of critique. Researchers who take the time and trouble to negotiate this complex and difficult theoretical terrain are usually staunch defenders. In fact, the main criticism that it has received in adolescent health research is that it has not been used enough. Froman and Owen (1991) suggests that the concept of self-efficacy might be useful in the study of everyday health-related behaviours during adolescence because of its prescriptive character and manipulable constructs. Although these are appealing features, the SCT is a demanding, complex theory that, up until now, has only exhibited modest predictive powers. According to Froman and Owen (1991), the measurement of self-efficacy is often reliable and valid. However, Sandberg, Rotheram-Borus, Bradley, and Martin (1988) found that adolescents' perception of self-efficacy in implementing HIV preventive behaviours was inconsistent across questionnaires, focus groups, and interviews. The fact remains that the SCT is a cognitively based theory that places behaviour in a chain-of-events model, and this may explain its apparently limited usefulness within adolescent populations.

Other social–cognitive approaches

There are several other social–cognitive theories used in health research and education, including Rotter's extension of the Social Learning theory, the locus of control construct (Rotter, 1966), theories related to self-perception (Bers, & Quinlan, 1992; de Maio Esteves, 1990), Self-Regulation theory (Becker, 1990), Self-Presentation theory (Koelen, 1988), Attribution theory (Lewis, & Daltroy, 1990), the Social Influences model (Perry, & Kelder, 1992) and the Life Skills approaches (Botvin, & Scheier, 1997). The Self-Presentation theory and the Social Influences model have shown some promising results in adolescent smoking and drug abuse prevention. Life Skills approaches, while generally less oriented towards exhuming behavioural determinants, have also been selectively effective. The locus of control construct from Rotter's work has been frequently utilised in adolescent health education and research.

Health locus of control is a generalised expectation about whether one's health is controlled by one's own behaviour (internal locus of control), or by forces external to oneself (external locus of control). Locus of control has often been subject to unwarranted comparison with self-efficacy. Bandura has illustrated the importance of making a distinction between the two constructs (Bandura, 1977a). While self-efficacy is behaviour and situation specific, locus of control is person specific, and resembles a trait. A person's belief concerning whether or not health is under personal behavioural control (locus of control) does not imply any particular convictions related to personal competence in the performance of any particular behaviour (self-efficacy).

Health locus of control is significantly related to adolescent health-related behaviour in approximately two-thirds of the studies in which it is measured. For instance, it has been significantly associated with suicidal behaviour (Pearce, & Martin, 1993), the ability to refuse a beer (Shope, Copeland, Mararg, Dielman, et al., 1993), contraceptive use (Sandler, Watson, & Levine, 1992), and smoking

(Eiser, Eiser, Gammage, & Morgan, 1989). Locus of control has shown no relationship to seat belt use (Desmond, Price, & O'Connell, 1985; Riccio-Howe, 1991), and weak predictive power for substance abuse in adolescent populations (Bearinger, & Blum, 1997).

The criticism of health locus of control in adolescent health research is primarily on methodological grounds. Adolescents' perception of locus of control has been found to be inconsistent across questionnaires, focus groups, and interviews (Sandberg et al., 1988). Age and gender differences found in adolescent health locus of control further complicate its use in health-related research (Cohen, Brownell, & Felix, 1990). In their review of the research, Giblin, Poland, and Ager (1988) question not only the reliability of self-report measures, but also the predictive value of health locus of control. While some of the correlational studies reviewed show significant relationships between locus of control and health behaviour, the predictive studies report predominantly non-significant contributions to the explanation of variance in health behaviours. Giblin and his colleagues offer several suggestions for enhancing health locus of control research, but five years after their first publication, they were forced to conclude that locus of control research in adolescent health had not improved (Giblin, 1992).

BELIEF-BASED APPROACHES

The Health Belief model

The Health Belief Model (HBM, Fig. 3.2) is, like the SCT, a value-expectancy theory (Becker, Drachman, & Kirscht, 1972; Rosenstock et al., 1988). It was developed around 1950 to explain widespread failure of the asymptomatic US population to accept disease preventatives or to undergo screening tests for conditions such as lung cancer (Godin, & Shepard, 1990). The HBM is based on the assumption that peoples' beliefs influence their behaviour. Beliefs carry evaluative meanings. The term 'belief' is used to refer to information that a person has about an object, behaviour, person, etc. This information may be factual, or a matter of opinion (Petty, & Cacioppo, 1981). Images of objects and behaviours, and representations of previous experiences with objects or behaviours, are also subsumed under the concept of beliefs (Eagly, & Chaiken, 1993).

In the original HBM, it was hypothesised that people would not perform preventive health behaviours unless they (1) possessed minimal levels of relevant health motivation and knowledge, (2) viewed themselves as potentially vulnerable to a relatively threatening condition, (3) were convinced of the effectiveness of the preventive behaviour, and (4) anticipated few difficulties in undertaking the recommended action.

The HBM has been modified and extended over the years to incorporate constructs from more recent theories. In the wake of the attitude theories which began to emerge decisively in the late 1960s, a measure of behavioural intentions

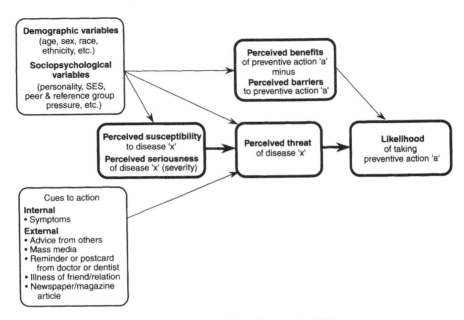

FIG. 3.2   Health Belief model (HBM) (adapted from Rosenstock, 1974).

is sometimes added to the HBM (Haefner, & Kirscht, 1970). Motivation, which was originally considered to be subsumed under perceived susceptibility and perceived severity, has occasionally been explicitly operationalised as 'salience of health as a value' (Mullen, Hersey, & Iverson, 1987). The publication of Bandura's seminal article on self-efficacy (Bandura, 1977a) also exerted some influence on the HBM. Concepts related to self-efficacy were originally considered to be incorporated in the perceived barriers construct of the HBM (Janz, & Becker, 1984). In 1988, Rosenstock, Strecher, and Becker argued persuasively for the addition of self-efficacy to the model as an autonomous construct (Rosenstock et al., 1988).

The HBM assumes that health is highly valued and that relevant cues, which stimulate health-related behaviours, are present. When these conditions are not met, the model may not be useful for, or relevant to, explaining behaviour (Becker, 1990). Since health is generally of low priority for adolescents (Spruijt-Metz, & Spruijt, 1997), these criteria could jeopardise the usefulness of the HBM for adolescent populations. While there has been some empirical support for the use of the HBM to explain adolescent health-related behaviours such as contraception use, likelihood to take preventive action against sexually transmitted disease, and dieting behaviours (Tappe, 1992), results of recent research has not been encouraging. In fact, Kirscht, in his review of the research, finds little support for the application of the HBM to health behaviour during youth (Kirscht, 1988). West, DuRant, and Pendergrast (1993) reported that adolescent compliance with dental appointments was not associated with any of the variables from the HBM. Hølund

(1990a, 1990b) found no connection between beliefs and behaviour in her study on sugar consumption in adolescence. Abraham, Sheeran, Spears, and Abrams (1992) found some support for the HBM in predicting HIV-preventive intentions in teenagers between the age of 16–18 years (17.8–24% of the variance in reported intentions was explained), but expressed their doubts about the adequacy of the HBM for explaining actual behaviour of adolescents. Petosa and Jackson (1991) found that the predictive power of the HBM for safer sex intentions among adolescents decreased dramatically with age. While the model accounted for a full 43% of the variance in intentions for seventh graders and 27% for ninth graders, the only significant predictor for the eleventh graders in their study was gender. These findings have been supported by several studies that show the HBM to be quite limited in its utility for predicting sexual practices in minority youth (Laraque, McLean, Brown-Peterside, & Ashton, 1997; Strack, Vincent, Hussey, & Kelly, 1998) and university students (Lollis, Johnson, & Antoni, 1997). Results of an HBM-based intervention aimed at preventing teenage pregnancy offered no support for the use of this theory (Eisen, Zellman, & McAlister, 1992).

One of the most thorough critiques of use of the HBM in adolescent populations, on both methodological and substantive grounds, is offered by Brown, DiClemente, and Reynolds (1991) in relation to HIV prevention. The methodological critique addresses the lack of reliability and validity of measures of various belief dimensions of the model, and the lack of empirically established relationships between the model's constructs. This makes it impossible to predict the extent of behavioural change that might follow by influencing one of the model's factors.

The theoretical critique is threefold. The first is that the HBM does not adequately address problems concerning maintenance of change in habitual behaviours. In this context, Brown, DiClemente, and Reynolds (1991) note that change and maintenance of recurrent behaviours relevant to HIV prevention are determined by complex interactions between adolescent and social environment. These interactions, based in cultural mores and norms, are beyond the theoretical reach of the HBM.

The second criticism concerns the lack of maturational constructs in the HBM, which are deemed necessary to assess influences of those cognitive and physical changes particular to adolescence. Different age groups within adolescence may require different models of behavioural change (Chapter 7). It has also been suggested that the adolescent's sense of invulnerability may distort their perception of susceptibility (Brown et al., 1991; Eklind, 1978). Research into unrealistic optimism has shown that people underestimate their personal susceptibility to health risks, and tend to think that the chance that any risky behaviour might lead to negative health outcomes is higher for others than for themselves (Jakobs, van Schie, Van Baaren, & van der Pligt, 1993). This would seriously limit the predictive powers of the HBM, as perceived susceptibility is one of the most important predictors of preventive health behaviour in the model. Biological factors, such as accelerated sexual maturation, in combination with cognitive factors, such as a lag in parallel changes in self-perceptions, may also influence risk perception.

The third theoretical criticism is that the HBM excludes peer group influence and emotional reactions. Although recent research has cast some doubt on the magnitude of peer influence upon health-related behaviours (Brown, DiClemente, & Park, 1992; Lau, Quadrel, & Hartman, 1990), the criticism concerning the exclusion of emotional reactions is in keeping with the theme of this review. Brown, DiClemente, and Reynolds (1991) note that the HBM is a rational-cognitive model, which implies a rational decision maker, and argue that adolescents are not so linear in logical formulation of problems and solutions. Their final recommendations include research into the diverse psychological purposes that risk taking might serve for adolescents, and assessment of the adolescents' perception of the world. They conclude that the HBM or any other model will be inadequate in adolescent health research without incorporation of comparable adolescent-specific factors.

Protection Motivation theory

The Protection Motivation theory (PMT) is a belief-based value-expectancy theory similar to the HBM, and it has its roots in drive-reduction models and attitude-persuasion theories (Eagly, & Chaiken, 1993). Drive-reduction models presume that fear and emotional tension have the functional properties of drives, which motivate responses, which in turn reduce fear and emotional tension. This reduction is inherently reinforcing, and any cognitive or behavioural response that contributes to or accompanies this reduction will thus be reinforced. Attitude theories assume that attitudes are prime determinants of behaviour, and persuasion theories are concerned with the nature of persuasive messages (definitions of attitudes can be found in the section discussing attitude-based theories, persuasion is touched on in the section on frameworks for multi-theoretical approaches). The PMT was originally designed to explain how people deal with the threat of danger and to explore the influence of threatening messages, or 'fear appeal communications', on human behaviour (Godin, & Shepard, 1990; Maddux, & Rogers, 1983; Rogers, 1983). According to the PMT, the emotional state of fear influences attitude and behaviour change indirectly through the appraisal of the severity of the danger. Although the PMT focuses on cognitively based mediating processes which are assumed to intervene between incoming information and behaviour, Rogers (1983) claims that it does not assume a purely rational decision maker because subjective heuristic judgements and subjectively appraised vividness of the sources of information are expected to bias appraisal processes. The PMT originally posited that the motivation to protect oneself depended upon (a) the perceived noxiousness or severity of the threatened event, (b) the perceived probability of the occurrence of the event (perceived susceptibility, danger, or vulnerability), and (c) the perceived effectiveness of the recommended preventive behaviour (perceived response efficacy) (Rogers, 1975). In 1983, three further conditions were added as prerequisites to protection motivation and preventive behaviour: (d) perceived self-efficacy to carry out the recommended preventive behaviour, (e) factors decreasing probability of risk behaviour must outweigh rewards associated with performance of risk behaviour, and (f) factors increasing probability of preventive behaviour must outweigh costs of preventive behaviour. In the preliminary research, self-efficacy proved to be a more powerful predictor of behaviour than any of the original constructs (Maddux, & Rogers, 1983), and it has since then been integrated into the theory. Figure 3.3 shows the PMT as Rogers envisioned it in 1983.

Results from the research conducted by Maddux and Rogers (1983) indicate that information about self-efficacy is more persuasive when people expect low

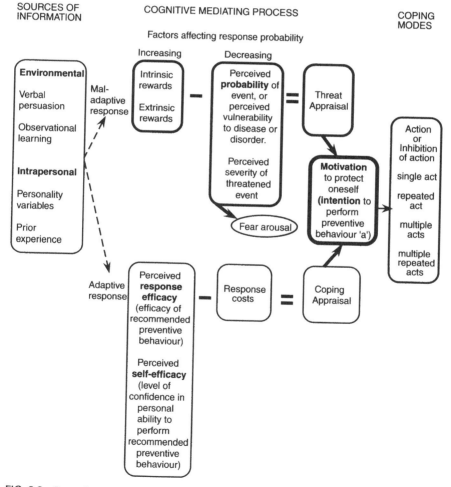

FIG. 3.3   Protection Motivation theory (PMT) (Adapted from Rogers, 1975. Revised version, Rogers, 1983; adapted from Maddux, & Rogers, 1983).

outcome efficacy than when they expect high outcome efficacy. Maddux and Rogers also found some interesting interactions between self-efficacy, outcome efficacy, and perceived susceptibility. When expectations of danger were low, but self-efficacy and outcome expectancies were high, people seemed to be persuaded to undertake preventive behaviour 'just in case', in what Maddux and Rogers (1983) term the 'precaution strategy'. When expectations of danger were high, however, either high self-efficacy or high response efficacy was enough to lead to intentions to adopt a preventive behaviour. In other words, if people feel threatened, and feel that they can successfully perform a preventive behaviour, they are likely to adopt it even if they are not particularly convinced that the behaviour will have a salutary effect. Maddux and Rogers called this the 'hyperdefensiveness strategy', which they conceded may be more directed towards reducing anxiety than towards avoiding danger. They observe that these strategies do not seem 'rational' or logical in the sense of traditional decision theories.

The PMT has not enjoyed wide use or support in adolescent health research. Ho (1992) did not find any relationships between the predictor variables and cigarette consumption in a study involving both adolescents and adults. In a Dutch study involving adolescents and adults, Bakker, Buunk, and Siero (1993) compared the adequacy of the PMT, the theory of Planned Behaviour (discussed below), and the HBM in predicting heterosexual's intentions to use condoms. The theory of Planned Behaviour fitted the data best, with the PMT running a close second. While neither response efficacy or response cost contributed to the equation, the PMT explained 36% of the variance in intentions to use condoms for the women and 43% for the men. These results must be viewed with caution for two reasons. In the first place, models that work for adults do not necessarily work for adolescents (Janz, & Becker, 1984; Kirscht, 1983) and although some adolescents participated in this research, the mean age of the sample was 31 years of age. In the second place, the relationship between intention to behave and actual behaviour is debatable. As mentioned earlier, this type of theory often predicts intentions better than it predicts actual behaviour (Eagly, & Chaiken, 1993; Kashima, Gallois, & McCamish, 1993).

Threat appeals may actually backfire when used in health education for children and adolescents. Using the cognitive fear-based approach of the PMT to disenfranchise tobacco use among 10–15-year-olds led to decreased intentions to refrain from tobacco use when the subjects did not believe that they could cope effectively with the danger presented in the appeals (Sturges, & Rogers, 1996).

In general, research has shown that the persuasive impact of fear tends to be stronger on attitudes and intentions than on behaviour itself. Rogers' original claim that severity, vulnerability, and response efficacy combined multiplicatively to influence intentions has not received any empirical support, nor has the interaction between threat and efficacy assumed in the 1983 version of the theory. The PMT and other drive-reduction theories do not shed any light on how the perception of threat might work to influence behaviour, or account for the possibility that threat information might bias or hinder cognitive processing. Eagly and Chaiken (1993) consider the most important contribution of this kind of drive-reduction model to be the proposition that the fear-persuasion relation can be understood by examining how fear arousal influences the cognitive processes that mediate acceptance of persuasive messages' recommendation. They put forward the Elaboration Likelihood model (discussed below) as a promising framework for further study of this proposition. In adolescent health research, the moral implications of using fear message must be weighed against the insufficient empirical support for the PMT and the degree of certainty about the actual health risks or benefits which can be attained by the behaviours to be addressed.

ATTITUDE-BASED APPROACHES

The theory of Reasoned Action

The theory of Reasoned Action (TRA) has been widely utilised in health behaviour research. The first version of this theory, the Behaviour Intention model, was published by Fishbein in 1967. The Behaviour Intention model was expanded and reintroduced as the theory of Reasoned Action in 1975 by Ajzen and Fishbein (see Fig. 3.4).

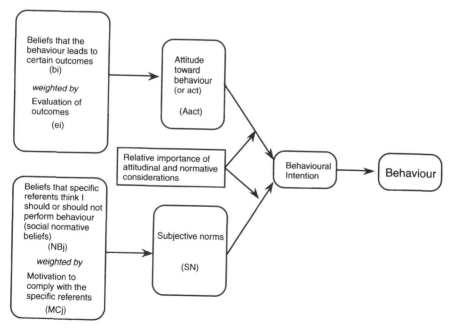

FIG. 3.4   Theory of Reasoned Action (TRA) (Adapted from Ajzen, & Fishbein, 1980).

According to the TRA, the sole direct determinant of behaviour is the intention to perform that behaviour. This theoretical unity between behaviour and intentions is based on the assumption (Ajzen, & Fishbein, 1980, p. 5) that "most actions of social relevance are under volitional control". Intentions are considered to be determined by (1) personal attitudes towards performing a specific behaviour (Aact) and (2) subjective norms (SN). In the TRA, attitudes toward a behaviour are measures of affective feelings toward that behaviour and do not directly include a cognitive or a behavioural component, as does the attitude construct defined by the Yale school (Rosenberg, & Hovland, 1960) and elaborated by Eagly and Chaiken (1993). In the TRA, the behavioural component is covered by the intentions construct, and the cognitive component by the beliefs (or expectancies) about behavioural outcomes (bi). Attitudes are determined by beliefs about behavioural outcomes (bi), which are weighted by the evaluation of these outcomes (ei). Here is an expectancy-value model. Attitude $= \Sigma$ Expectancy $\times$ Value for each attribute of the object in question (Eagly, & Chaiken, 1993, p. 106). Subjective norms (SN) are measures of the perceived feelings of important others in general about the subject undertaking the performance of a behaviour. Social normative beliefs (NBj) are measures of the perceived feelings of specific important others about the subject undertaking the performance of a behaviour, and are weighted by the motivation to comply with the specific referents (MCj). Subjective norms mediate the effect of social normative beliefs upon behavioural intentions (Ajzen, & Fishbein, 1980; van den Putte, 1993).

Several modifications of the TRA have been attempted. In 1977, Triandis introduced his theory of Interpersonal Behaviour. This theory is very similar to the TRA, although due to the inclusion of habit (or past behaviour), skills, and other vital constructs which generate distinctive interactions and weights, it cannot simply be considered a modification of the theory (Fig. 3.5).

In the theory of Interpersonal Behaviour, the influence of habit or past behaviour, and the influence of personal norms are included. Personal normative beliefs are the respondent's personal feelings about whether or not they should engage in a particular behaviour, weighted by motivation to comply with themselves. Ajzen and Fishbein had originally included personal normative beliefs in their model, but dropped them from the final version because they found them empirically indistinguishable from intentions (van den Putte, 1993). While Triandis' model has often yielded more accurate predictions of behaviour than the TRA (Boyd, & Wandersman, 1991; Godin, & Shepard, 1986; Siebold, & Roper, 1979; Valois, Desharnais, & Godin, 1988), the explanatory power of personal normative beliefs is usually minimal (explaining an average of 3% of variance in intentions) (van den Putte, 1993). In 1979, Bentler and Speckart (Bentler, & Speckart, 1979) added past behaviour directly to the TRA. They also posited a direct influence of attitude on behaviour, as have several other authors (Bentler, & Speckart, 1981; Manstead, Proffitt, & Smart, 1983; van den Putte, 1993). The model proposed by Bentler and Speckart is shown in Fig. 3.6.

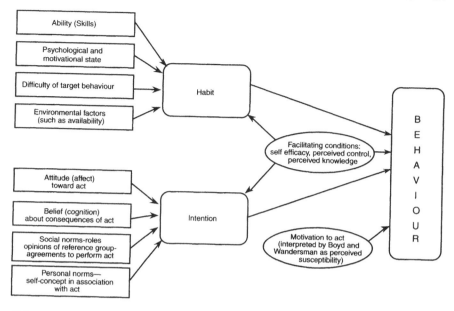

FIG. 3.5   Theory of Interpersonal Behaviour (TIB). (Triandis, 1977. Adapted from Siebold, & Roper, 1979; Godin, & Shepard, 1990).

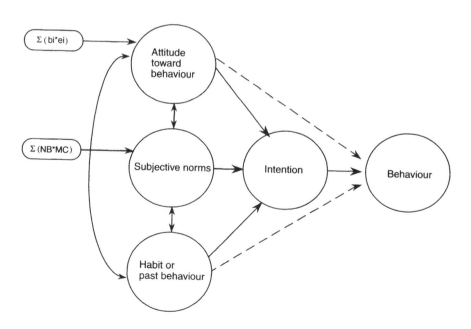

FIG. 3.6   Theory of Reasoned Action (TRA) plus Bentler and Speckart's additions (Adapted from Bentler, & Speckart, 1979).

A non-trivial portion of behavioural variance was predicted from previous behaviour and attitudes, with the effects of intentions partialled out. The hypothesis that behaviour is predominantly premeditated and only indirectly influenced by non-cognitive elements was refuted, although several statistical artefacts were later detected in the assessments of the direct influence of attitude upon behaviour (van den Putte, 1993). Previous behaviour, sometimes appearing as experience or habit, has remained a popular addition to the TRA (Godin, & Shepard, 1990; Kashima et al., 1993; Stacy et al., 1994). The self-efficacy construct has also been used in conjunction with the TRA or reduced versions of the TRA. Research with this 'Attitude—Social Norms—Self-Efficacy' model (ASE), based on the TRA, the SCT, and McGuire's model of behavioural change (McGuire, 1985), shows that self-efficacy provides a unique contribution to the prediction of behavioural intentions consistent with the magnitude indicated in the above section on the SCT (Basen-Engquist, & Parcel, 1992; de Vries et al., 1988; Kok et al., 1991).

The TRA has been used in adolescent health research, most frequently in the study of condom, drug, alcohol, and tobacco use. The TRA accounted for 10.6% of the variance in intentions to use condoms and 14.4% of the variance in condom use in a population of Texas ninth-graders (Basen-Engquist, & Parcel, 1992). In a study of drug and alcohol use under Midwest senior high-school students in the USA, between 12% and 20% of the variance in behaviour was accounted for by attitude and social norms (Laflin, Moore-Hirschl, Weis, & Hayes, 1994). One study looked at the predictive power of the TRA for condom use and number of sexual partners in three samples: early adolescents, late adolescents, and college students. The attitude construct contributed to the prediction of condom use in all three samples. None of the constructs in the TRA could predict number of sexual partners in the two adolescent samples (Serovich, & Greene, 1997). Past behaviour has been included in several studies of condom use in both college and high-school populations. Kashima et al. (1993) found that when behaviour conditions including the availability of a condom and an agreement with the partner to use it were satisfied, intention interacted with past behaviour to predict actual behaviour in a population of college students between the ages of 17 and 21. Brown et al. (1992) found that past behaviour was predictive of condom use in the study of ninth, tenth, and eleventh graders in Rhode Island. They also found that the perception of condom use as normative to their peer group was related to behavioural intentions but not to actual behaviour. This contributes to the growing evidence that subjective norms in the form of peer influence may not play the decisive role in adolescent health-related behaviour that it has long been accorded (Lau et al., 1990). It must be added that most of the research supporting moderate to low effects of peer influence on health-related behaviours has *not* been done in the poorer areas of England or the ghettos of America, where much of the early research on peer influence in adolescence originated (Coleman, & Hendry, 1990). The major differences in health and health behaviours related to socio-economic differences indicate that different determinants are at work in different SES groups

(Mackenbach, 1992; Spruijt-Metz, 1998a; Wilson et al., 1997b). In this context, it is important to note that the predictive power of the TRA depends upon the identification of all or most of the outcomes and beliefs that are salient to the target population, and these may differ across subgroups of the population. It has therefore been suggested that more rigorous preliminary data collection is demanded than has previously been indicated (Carter, 1990).

Although the TRA and other attitude-based models are of considerable value in health research, they have received relevant criticism. The major critiques of the TRA are important for adolescent health-related research as well as for health research in general. They include the lack of a self-efficacy type construct and the fact that the assumption upon which the model is based is often not met: most behaviour is not under total volitional control (Carter, 1990). The assumption of volitional control is illustrative of the assumptions of a rational person and the chain-of-events model of behaviour, and is subject to the objections that have been raised in their context. Moreover, the degree of behavioural control depends on many personal variables, such as skills and knowledge, as well as external variables, such as availability of resources. The degree to which behaviours are considered to be under volitional control also varies depending upon the degree to which the tenets of Freudian theories of the unconscious are sustained and the influences of family, friends, institutions, authority figures, the media, and many other sources upon behaviour are recognised. Methodological discussions of the research done with the TRA and other attitude theories often focus on the correspondence, or lack of it, between the attitude and behaviour measurements with respect to specific actions and targets (Ajzen, & Fishbein, 1977). An important criticism of the use of TRA and all value-expectancy models for adolescent populations is that they are rational approaches to behaviour, assuming a rational, logical, motivated decision maker in a chain-of-events framework which does not take the adolescent into account (Spruijt-Metz, 1995, 1997, 1998a). Perhaps the most salient criticism of the use of attitude theories in adolescent health research was offered by Ajzen himself. During adolescence, many attitudes relevant to health-related behaviours are in formative stages, and are usually unstable and malleable. However, in order to be useful in the prediction of intentions and behaviour, attitudes need to be fairly stable (Ajzen, 1994; Eagly, & Chaiken, 1993).

The theory of Planned Behaviour

In the wake of the above mentioned general critique and the popularity of Bandura's work, Ajzen (1985) introduced an extended version of the TRA in 1985, the theory of Planned Behaviour (TPB). This model adds the construct of perceived behavioural control to the TRA. The 1985 TPB included constructs concerning the strength of a person's attempt to perform a given behaviour, but the simplified version introduced by Ajzen and Madden in 1986 (Fig. 3.7) has received more attention and will be addressed here.

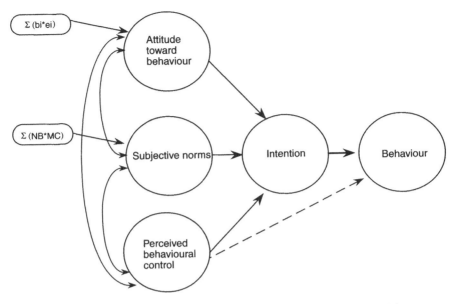

FIG. 3.7   Theory of Planned Behaviour (TBP) (Adapted from Ajzen, & Madden, 1986).

Perceived behavioural control includes perceived presence or absence of requisite resources, opportunities, skills, knowledge, time, a workable plan, money, willpower, etc (Ajzen, & Madden, 1986; Becker, 1990). Perceived behavioural control is presumed to subsume the effects of past behaviour as well as the constructs of self-efficacy and locus of control (Ajzen, & Madden, 1986). It has also been suggested that perceived behavioural control subsumes the construct of perceived barriers to action (Godin, & Shepard, 1990).

The power of the TPB did not exceed that of the TRA in predicting Midwest American high school students' use of drugs and alcohol (Laflin et al., 1994) although it must be said that this study employed a broad concept of self-esteem rather than the narrower construct of perceived behavioural control. Rannie and Craig (1997) conducted rigorous qualitative preliminary studies to ascertain salient beliefs before assessing the relationships between constructs from the TPB and adolescent girls' attitudes toward and intentions to carry out condom use. The model accounted for 50% of the variance in intentions to use condoms, which is substantial. However, the caveat concerning the precarious relationship between intentions and behaviour remains in place. The TPB did provide interesting results in a theory-based intervention on the practice of testicular self-examination by high-school males (Murphy, & Brubaker, 1990). In this study, one group received an informational message, one a theory-based message, and there was one control group. At the time of the intervention, the three variables, attitude towards the behaviour, subjective norm, and perceived behavioural control, explained 35% of the variance in intentions to perform testicular self-examination. However, only attitude contributed significantly to the equation. At the follow-up conducted one month later, 42% of the group that received the theory-based message reported performing testicular self-examination, as compared to 23% in the informational message group and 6% in the control group. However, it was found that the only significant difference between the groups was in intentions to conduct testicular self-examination in the future. They did not differ in attitude towards the behaviour, perceived behavioural control, or subjective norms. The theory-based message was the most effective, but the theoretical model does not adequately explain its effectiveness. These results are characteristic of the mixed and sometimes difficult to interpret results often attained when general attitude models are used for research in adolescent populations.

THEORIES OF ADOLESCENT HEALTH-RELATED BEHAVIOUR

To gain a greater understanding of adolescent health-related behaviour, several researchers have generated models specifically for this purpose, including maturational concepts and cognitive constructs particular to adolescents, and borrowing the most viable constructs from extant social–cognitive, belief-based, and attitude-based theories and models. Jessor's Problem Behaviour theory (Jessor, 1984) focuses primarily on risk behaviour and has received the most research, and Tappe's model of Personal Investment (Tappe, 1992) offers promising new insights into adolescent health behaviour. These two models will be reviewed here. Langer and Warheit's (1992) Pre-Adult Health Decision-Making model combines sociological, developmental, social interactional, and decision process elements. Although it will not be reviewed here due to the lack of empirical research that has been conducted using this model, it deserves mention as one of the theories developed specifically to understand adolescent health behaviour.

The Problem Behaviour theory

Jessor's Problem Behaviour theory (PBT) (Jessor, 1984) was originally developed in 1968 to guide in the study of adolescent deviance in the southwestern United States. Jessor found that a subset of problem behaviours—behaviours that constitute transgressions of societal and/or legal norms and that tend to elicit some sort of social control response—such as drug abuse, alcohol abuse, suicide attempts, unprotected sex, and smoking, were linked and tended to covary systematically in adolescent populations. The PBT was developed to explain adolescent participation in such problem behaviours. He posited that these seemingly different behaviours may all serve a similar social-psychological function: overt repudiation of conventional norms or expression of independence from parental control. Over the years, the PBT has been modified to accommodate cross-cultural (Organista,

Chun, & Marín, 1998) and longitudinal studies of problem behaviours (Jessor, 1998), and has also been applied to the study of health-enhancing behaviours in adolescence (Donovan, Jessor, & Costa, 1993). The point of departure of the PBT is the assumption of three major systems and fluctuating social-psychological relationships between them. These systems are the personality system, the perceived environment system, and the behaviour system (see Fig. 3.8).

Within each system, the interrelation of the variables can lead to a dynamic state called proneness, which in turn can lead to likelihood of problem behaviour, in this case health-risk behaviour. This means that it is possible to refer to personality proneness, environmental proneness, behavioural proneness, and to their combination, termed psychosocial proneness, toward problem behaviour. The concept of psychosocial proneness is the key theoretical basis for predicting and explaining variations in adolescent problem behaviour. The behaviour system includes two structures that indicate the two possible outcomes depending upon the degree of proneness: problem behaviour structure and conventional behaviour structure. Problem behaviour has been defined. Conventional behaviours are socially approved, normatively expected, and institutionalised as appropriate behaviours for adolescents. Examples of conventional behaviours given by Jessor are involvement in scholastic and religious activities. According to Jessor, the dimension underlying psychosocial proneness and proneness in the three separate systems can best be termed conventionality–unconventionality. Variation along this continuum accounts for proneness, which in turn accounts for variation in problem behaviour in adolescence (Jessor, 1984).

The PBT has not, as such, undergone many changes since 1984. Rather, the area of research has been expanded to include hypotheses concerning the buffering effects of conventionality factors (Jessor, 1991, 1993), assessment and identification of protective factors (Jessor, 1998) and the explanatory power of conventionality for health behaviour (Chewning, & Van Koningsveld, 1998; Costa, Jessor, Fortenberry, & Donovan, 1996; Donovan, Jessor, & Costa, 1991; Donovan et al., 1993).

The PBT generally explains between one-third to one-half of the variance in problem behaviours in populations of American adolescents (Donovan et al., 1991; Jessor, 1984). In one extensive study, the PBT model was used to predict adolescent every-day health behaviours including exercise, sleep, seat belt use, attention to healthy diet, and healthy food preferences (Donovan et al., 1991). Conventionality–unconventionality predicted between 3% to 14% of the variance in health behaviours. This cannot be considered impressive, due to the number of variables that were measured and included in the equation to obtain this result. The PBT has repeatedly been used to research what has come to be considered a health behaviour (condom use) (Basen-Engquist, Edmundson, & Parcel, 1996; Chewning, & Van Koningsveld, 1998; Costa et al., 1996). Most of the results from this research suggest that the PBT needs further adaptation for use in the study of health behaviours (Basen-Engquist et al., 1996; Chewning, & Van Koningsveld, 1998). The model does not perform consistently over different behaviours and samples.

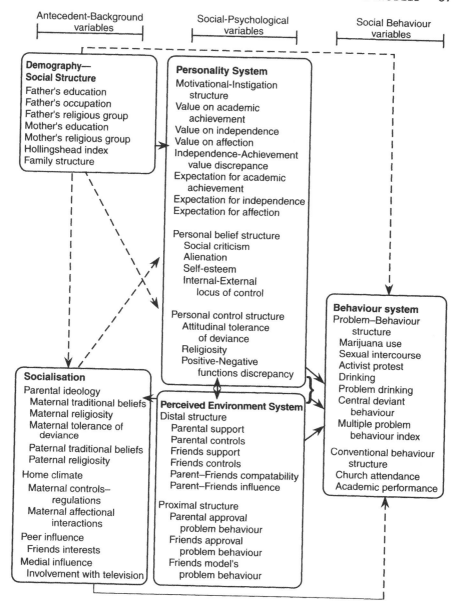

FIG. 3.8   Problem Behaviour theory (PBT) (Jessor & Jessor, 1977). Copyright © (1977) Academic Press. Reprinted with permission.

Jessor and his team have contributed immensely to the theoretical and methodological discussion of adolescent health and risk behaviour. The PBT has proven useful in understanding adolescent risk behaviours and indicates a number of possible targets for intervention, although it is not specifically prescriptive. The usefulness of the PBT for understanding adolescent health behaviour appears to be limited, perhaps partially due to the fact that health behaviours do not form a coherent, interrelated whole as do problem behaviours (Donovan et al., 1991, 1993; Spruijt-Metz, & Spruijt, 1996). One of the underlying assumptions in Jessor's PBT is that risk behaviours all serve similar psychological functions, or have similar personal meanings. Because he was investigating highly correlated problem behaviours, one group of related psychological functions seemed to have been sufficient and workable. However, one set of psychological functions might not be able to describe how adolescents perceive health-enhancing behaviours because this group of behaviours does not correlate or form interpretable factors. These distinctions may account for the fact that the PBT has been less successful in describing and predicting health-related behaviours (Donovan et al., 1991, 1993).

The main criticism of the PBT is its lack of parsimony. Using the PBT requires use of long questionnaires in order to include all the constructs, which can be fatiguing for the subjects. It also requires large populations in order to allow for analysis of so many constructs, which are not always available and can lead to significant findings with little or no relevance (very small effect sizes; Cohen, 1988). Lastly, the inclusion of so many unmanipulable constructs practically excludes experimental research, thus limiting the possibilities of testing the theory fully.

The model of Personal Investment

The model of Personal Investment (MPI) (Tappe, 1992) is based on Maehr and Braskamp's (1986) theory of Personal Investment, and was developed specifically to explain adolescent health-enhancing behaviour. Tappe integrates insights gained in her earlier research on adolescent health behaviour, Maehr and Breskamp's theory, and constructs from many of the theories reviewed here into her model (Fig. 3.9).

The subjective meaning of behaviour, which is the product of interactions between factors related to the person, the environment, and the behaviour, is proposed as the critical determinant of adolescents' health-related behaviour. This meaning is composed of six interrelated components: (1) sense of self perceptions, (2) personal incentives, (3) perceived barriers, (4) perceived options, (5) perceived situational opportunities, and (6) perceived situational climate. These six components determine the subjective meaning, which in turn determines behaviour. Subjective meaning is considered a motivational determinant of behaviour, making Tappe's theory the only one in this review that is grounded in motivation theories of behaviour. She does not only attempt to describe the mechanisms that govern behaviour, but also the motivations that lead to behaviour.

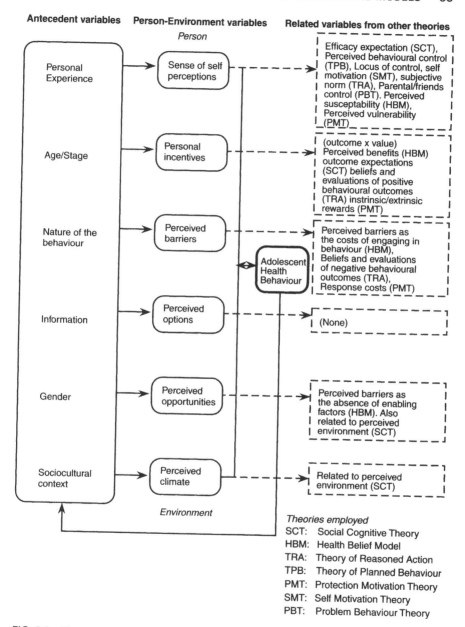

FIG. 3.9   The model of Personal Investment (MPI) (Adapted from Tappe, 1992).

The MPI has not yet been tested empirically in its full form. Research testing components of the model has, however, been conducted. Tappe, Duda, and Menges-Ehrnwald (1990) found that personal incentives, perceptions of sense of self, and perceived options accounted for 19% of the variance in exercise behaviour in an American male adolescent population, and 25% of the variance in exercise behaviour in an American female adolescent population. The same three variables contributed significantly to the prediction of adherence to athletic injury rehabilitation regimes in a population of college athletes (Duda, Smart, & Tappe, 1989)

A comprehensive report on the weaknesses of the MPI has been provided by Tappe herself (Tappe, 1992). The main criticisms concern the emphasis on the belief-behaviour relationship and rational decision-making processes, failure to fully address the influence of emotions upon health-related behaviour, the use of nascent constructs which have not yet shown predictive validity, and the methodological difficulties involved in measuring and testing such a large model. Another criticism of the model has to do with the differential strength of intrinsic versus extrinsic motivators. The personal incentive construct, which is defined as the reasons why adolescents engage in a given health-related behaviour, does not account for the possibility that intrinsic incentives with which adolescents imbue behaviours may be more influential for behaviour than any extrinsic incentive (Spruijt-Metz, 1995; see also Chapter 8 of this book). Tappe's adherence to the value-expectancy tradition impedes the investigation of the central concepts in the theory: the meaning which behaviours assume in the minds of the adolescents, and the degree to which these private, personal meanings influence behaviour. Tappe concluded that the final model did not fully account for the less rational and less linear aspects of adolescent health behaviour. Nevertheless, in the opinion of this author Tappe has done adolescent health researchers a great service by attempting an integration of several prominent theoretical schools with the exclusive goal of understanding adolescent health behaviour.

FRAMEWORKS FOR MULTI-THEORETICAL APPROACHES

This veritable inundation of available theories leaves health researchers to choose one of several possible courses of action. The most obvious course of action is to choose from the available theories in accordance with the settings, subjects, and behaviours of interest. In view of the percentage of explained variance that the available theories have generally achieved, a second course of action would be to develop new constructs or theories to improve explanatory power. This possibility will be addressed in the conclusion of this chapter. A third possible course of action is to attempt a relevant and workable integration of several theories, as Tappe has done. A fourth possible course of action will be addressed in this section: the use of one of the extant frameworks for multi-theoretical approaches. These frameworks attempt to cut across existing theories and offer general theories of change which can either be used within other theories, to unite several theories, or to indicate which theories might be most appropriate for which behaviours at which point in the change process. Two of these frameworks will be reviewed here: Petty and

Cacioppo's Elaboration Likelihood model, and Prochaska and DiClemente's Transtheoretical model.

The Elaboration Likelihood model

The Elaboration Likelihood model (ELM) was introduced in 1981 (Petty, & Cacioppo, 1981). It has its roots in attitude and persuasion research, and attempts to explain the mechanisms governing attitude formation and change. Because most of the theories that assume relationships between attitude and behaviour do not explore the actual mechanisms involved in attitude formation, the ELM could conceivably be used in conjunction with any of them to improve both explanatory and prescriptive powers. The ELM also provides a context for consideration of attribution approaches and social judgement theory, neither of which have enjoyed much exploration for their possible relevance to adolescent health research and education (Eagly, & Chaiken, 1993). Petty and Cacioppo belong to the school of attitude theorists that envision attitude as being comprised of cognitive, behavioural, and affective elements, which can initiate or influence cognitive, behavioural, and affective processes of change. The ELM is based on the premise that persuasion leads to attitude change (and assumes afterwards that attitude has to do with behaviour, but the specifics of that relationship will depend on the chosen theory of behaviour change). Petty and Cacioppo specify two qualitatively different routes to persuasion and claim that most attitude theories can be viewed as an example of one or the other. Theories emphasising the mediational importance of argument-based thinking represent the central route to attitude change, and theories that specify psychological mechanisms that do not include argument processing represent the peripheral route to attitude change. Central to the ELM is the construct termed 'argument quality'. This refers to the recipient's perception that a message is comprised of strong and convincing arguments as opposed to weak and specious ones. Strong messages elicit favourable thoughts about the message's advocated position, weak messages elicit unfavourable thoughts about that position. Table 3.1 gives the seven postulates of the ELM as presented by Petty and Cacioppo (1986)

The term elaboration refers to the extent to which people think about issue-relevant arguments contained in persuasive messages. When situational and individual variables allow for high motivation and the ability for issue-relevant thinking, elaboration likelihood is said to be high. Peripheral cues are variables capable of affecting persuasion without affecting argument scrutiny. The main hypothesis of the ELM is that elaboration likelihood mediates the route to persuasion. When motivation and ability for elaboration are high, the central route will be followed. When motivation and ability are low, the peripheral route will be followed (Eagly, & Chaiken, 1993; Pearce, & Martin, 1993; Petty, & Cacioppo, 1981, 1986). Attitude changes that result from central route processing will be more persistent, predict behaviour better, and be more resistant to counterpersuasion than

TABLE 3.1

Postulates of the Elaboration Likelihood model

1. People are motivated to hold correct attitudes.
2. Although people want to hold correct attitudes, the amount and nature of issue-relevant elaboration in which people are willing or able to engage to evaluate a message vary with individual and situational factors.
3. Variables can affect the amount and direction of attitude change by (A) serving as persuasive arguments, (B) serving as peripheral cues, and/or (C) affecting the extent or direction of issue and argument elaboration.
4. Variables affecting motivation and/or ability to process a message in a relatively objective manner can do so by either enhancing or reducing argument scrutiny.
5. As motivation and/or ability to process arguments is decreased, peripheral cues become relatively more important determinants of persuasion. Conversely, as argument scrutiny is increased, peripheral cues become relatively less important determinants of persuasion.
6. Variables affecting message processing in a relatively biased manner can produce either a positive (favourable) or negative (unfavourable) motivational and/or ability bias to the issue-relevant thoughts attempted.
7. Attitude changes that result mostly from processing issue-relevant arguments (central route) will show greater temporal persistence, greater prediction of behaviour, and greater resistance to counterpersuasion than attitude changes that result mostly from peripheral cues.

(Eagly, & Chaiken, 1993, p. 307). Copyright © (1993) Academic Press.
Reprinted with permission.

changes attained by way of the peripheral route. Figure 3.10 shows the antecedents and consequents of the two routes to persuasion.

The ELM has not been used a great deal in adolescent health research. General research on the ELM has supported the prediction that the quality of argumentation influences attitude more when recipients are highly motivated and/or capable of elaborative processing. The hypothesised persistence and predictive powers of attitudes formed via the central route have also received empirical support (Eagly, & Chaiken, 1993). The usefulness of the ELM in health-related research with American college student populations has received some support in areas such as substance abuse prevention (Scott, & Ambroson, 1994), AIDS prevention (Flora, & Maibach, 1990), and treatment of eating disorders (Neimeyer, Guy, & Metzler, 1989).

Criticism of the ELM is that it is descriptive rather than explanatory. Petty and Cacioppo caution that the model does not indicate why arguments are considered strong or weak, why some variables serve as peripheral cues, or why some variables affect information processing (Petty, & Cacioppo, 1986). Eagly and Chaiken's (1993) main criticisms of the model are that, while the model predicts that peripheral cues will have little impact when elaboration likelihood is high, it does not explain why this should be so, nor does it specify the mechanisms that govern peripheral route persuasion and attitude change. The model has several attractive features. One is that it takes objective knowledge and skills into account. Another is that it deals specifically with attitude formation, which is part and parcel of the

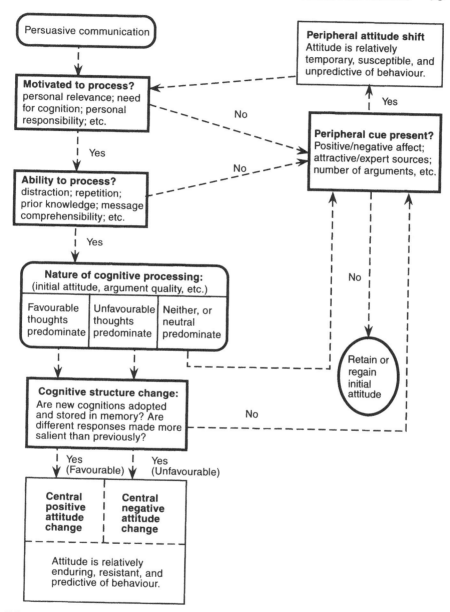

FIG. 3.10   The Elaboration Likelihood model of attitude change (ELM) (Petty, & Cacioppo, 1981, 1986). Copyright © (1986) Academic Press. Reprinted with permission.

developmental process in the adolescent years (Cobb, 1998). The central route describes rational processes, but the peripheral route leaves room for a less rational model of behaviour.

The Transtheoretical model

The last theory to be addressed in this review is Prochaska and DiClemente's Transtheoretical model (TM) (Prochaska, & DiClemente, 1983; Prochaska et al., 1994). Prochaska and DiClemente base their model on their observations that people appear to go through similar stages of change no matter what kind of psychotherapy they undergo. Although the TM was originally developed to explain processes which take place in the course of psychotherapy, it has since been applied to many health-related behaviours (Prochaska et al., 1994). The TM has two basic dimensions: stages of change and processes of change. Stages refer to an orderly sequence of changes through which people pass. Some people move faster than others do, and some might stabilise for long periods at one stage, but the order is assumed and no stage is skipped. Processes of change refer to different techniques or intervention approaches. Figure 3.11 shows the five stages of change and the ten processes of change which comprise the TM.

The TM not only implies that different intervention approaches are needed at different stages of change, but also suggests which processes of change will be most effective at each stage. Many of the processes identified in the TM can be related to constructs from other models, and research continues to be done on integrating constructs from decision theories (Janis, & Mann, 1977), the SCT (Velicer, DiClemente, Rossi, & Prochaska, 1990), the HBM (Strecher et al., 1994), and other by now familiar theories. Measures of pros and cons associated with target behaviours and a decisional balance measurement (derived from the pros and cons) is often used in conjunction with the model, as is the self-efficacy construct (Grimley, & Lee, 1997; Grimley, Riley, Bellis, & Prochaska, 1993; Prochaska et al., 1994; Velicer, Prochaska, Fava, Norman, & Redding, 1998)

Prochaska et al. (1994) studied 12 health-related behaviours, including weight control, high fat diets, safe sex, and delinquent behaviour. Only the delinquent group was made up of adolescent subjects. The safe sex, high fat, and weight control groups were college students. The other eight behaviours were studied in older populations. For all the behaviours studied, the cons (or disadvantages, barriers, and so forth) of changing behaviours were salient in the stages before action, and a cross-over to salience of the pros (or advantages, rewards, and so forth) of behavioural change prefaced transition into the action stage. In a following study, Prochaska et al. (1994) found that a 0.5 standard deviation decrease in cons and a 1.0 standard deviation increase in pros precipitated the progression from precontemplation to contemplation and from contemplation to action stages of behavioural change. Pros and cons were found to be related to stages of change for both contraceptive and condom use in a population of American college students (Grimley et al., 1993). Support for the stages of change has also been found in research in adult populations in The Netherlands (de Vries, & Backbier, 1995). Preliminary support has been furnished for the TM as a descriptive and diagnostic tool for the prevention of smoking (Wang, Fitzhugh, Eddy, & Westerfield, 1996),

(Motivational) Stages of Change

Precontemplation
Not interested in behaviour change
Contemplation
Thinking about changing in the future
Preparation
Getting ready to change soon
Action
The first 0–6 months of change
Maintenance/relapse
After 6 months of successful change OR relapse.

Constructs integrated from other models:

From Self-Efficacy Theory
(Velicer, DiClemente, Rossi, & Prochaska, 1990)
Temptations
Cognitions involving temptation to relapse to old behaviour
Confidence
Cognitions of confidence in one's ability to carry out and maintain new behaviour

From Janis & Mann's (1977) Decision-Making Model
(Prochaska, Velicer, Rossi, Goldstein, Marcus, Rakowski, Fiore, Harlow, Redding, Rosenbloom, & Rossi, 1994)
Pros (prevalent in action phase)
Advantages of desired behaviour
Cons (prevalent in precontemplation stage)
Disadvantages of desired behaviour

10 Processes of Change
5 cognitive processes:
(Used most during precontemplation and contemplation)
Consciousness raising
Open to change: Read about, think about, talk about relevant behaviour change
Dramatic relief
Emotionally moved by realisation that behaviour can be harmful
Environmental re-evaluation
Realisation that undesired behaviour has negative consequences for environment
Social liberation
Realisation that, for instance, smoking is forbidden in many public places
Self-re-evaluation
Changing self-image from someone who performs undesired behaviour to someone who performs desired behaviour

5 behavioural processes:
(Used most during action and maintenance)
Self-liberation
Acquiring the feeling that one has control over one's behaviour
Stimulus control
Correction of environment, such as removing ashtrays, sweets, fatty foods
Reinforcement management
Rewarding oneself for positive behaviour, expecting compliments from others
Counter conditioning
Replacing undesired behaviour with desired behaviour
Helping relationships
Expected social support for positive change

FIG. 3.11   Transtheoretical Model (TM) (Adapted from Prochaska & DiClemente, 1983; Prochaska et al., 1994).

the promotion of exercise (Nigg, & Courneya, 1998) and condom use (Grimley, & Lee, 1997) in adolescent populations.

De Vries and Backbier (1995) have given a thorough critique of the TM. They note that the TM enriches previous theories by positing that formation and change of cognition and behaviour is mediated by processes, and that certain processes are more appropriate for certain motivational stadia. These demarcations can be of great value in understanding behaviour and creating effective health education for different populations. However, the model does not explain why certain processes are more appropriate at certain motivational stadia. Furthermore, they stress the need for research into the place of attitudes, self-efficacy, and social norms within the TM framework, and the exact implications of stage-specific processes for health education. The TM has yet to be extensively tried out in adolescent health-related research. Its usefulness may be limited due to the fact that most adolescents must be considered to be precontemplators in relation to most health-enhancing behaviours (Spruijt-Metz, & Spruijt, 1997). As the literature reviewed here suggests, this may not be the case where problem behaviours such as unsafe sex, drug, cigarette, and alcohol use are concerned. The prescriptive character of the TM and blueprint it offers for the integration of other theories makes the TM promising, although it must be cautioned that the TM is not usually fully tested (Kaplan, Sallis, & Patterson, 1993). One of the main drawbacks of the TM for use with adolescent populations is that it remains an essentially rational model, leaving limited room for the adolescents' perception of the world in a broader sense.

CONCLUSIONS

Five categories of theories have been reviewed: social–cognitive, belief-based, attitude-based, theories directed explicitly towards the understanding of adolescent health-related behaviour, and multi-theoretical frameworks. These theories are designed to describe, predict, and eventually offer the possibility of manipulating behaviour. How useful are they in general for adolescent health-related research and education? Let us have another look at the six criteria for a 'good theory' listed at the beginning of this chapter and try to judge the theories presented here within that framework (Table 3.2).

A distinctly mottled picture appears, with some theories doing well on some criteria some of the time. Most of the theories fail to meet criterion 1, which is usually considered the most important criterion for a theory that claims to explain behaviour. The theories specifically developed to understand adolescent health-related behaviour could be expected to perform better in adolescent populations, and that is indeed the case with the Problem Behaviour theory and the model of Personal Investment. However, these models fail to meet the fourth, fifth, and sixth criteria, and are only moderately successful on the second criterion.

I had originally embarked upon this extensive review of the literature in order to be able to make an informed choice of theory upon which to base my ensuing research and interventions. However, at the end of the journey, none of the theories seemed to describe and predict adolescent health-related behaviour in a satisfactory manner. As I delved deeper into the literature, the third criterion—relevance to the target group—became more of an issue. Looking at Table 3.2, most of the theories reviewed here seem to fail to fulfil that criterion. This conclusion must be reached judging by the modest descriptive and predictive powers the theories retain for adolescent health-related behaviours. The theories specifically developed for adolescents fare better in this respect, but the Problem Behaviour theory is less useful in describing healthy behaviours, and the model of Personal Investment seems quite unwieldy for use in the field.

Where do the major theoretical frameworks seem to fail in adolescent research? The answer might lie in their failure to accommodate major developmental issues

TABLE 3.2

Six criteria for a 'good theory' for adolescent health education and research

	Criterion 1 Describes and predicts adolescent health behaviour	Criterion 2 Prescriptive potential for behaviour change	Criterion 3 Relevant for the target group	Criterion 4 Empirically testable	Criterion 5 Parsimonious	Criterion 6 User-friendly
Social cognitive theory	Modest	Yes	?	Problematic	No	No
Locus of control	Mediocre	No	?	Problematic	Yes	No
Health belief model	Modest	Moderate	No	Yes	Depends	Moderate
Protection motivation theory	Modest	Moderate	No	Yes	Depends	Moderate
Theory of reasoned action	Fluctuates: better with "past behaviour" added	Moderate	No	Yes	Depends	Yes
Theory of planned behaviour	Mixed	Moderate	No	Yes	Depends	Yes
Problem behaviour theory	Good (problem behaviour) Modest (health behaviour)	Moderate	Yes	No	No	No
Model of personal investment	Good	Moderate	Yes	No	No	No
Elaboration likelihood model	Mixed, needs more research	Yes	?	Problematic	No	No
Transtheoretical model	Preliminary support for some behaviours	Yes	?	Yes	No	Yes

in adolescence. To return to the *Leitmotiv* of this review, many of these theories and models represent rational approaches to behaviour, assuming rational people who understand cause and effect in a linear fashion and base their reasonable and autonomous decisions on available information. This model of human behaviour places a rational person at the centre of a network of lines and arrows that guide us neatly through pathways of logically connected constructs such as attitudes, intentions, beliefs, and knowledge, and inevitably lead us to behaviour in a linear fashion. In these theories and models, much is missing of what we know about adolescents' perceptual image of the world (Brown et al., 1991). This may explain their limited descriptive powers within adolescent populations. They do not seem to be able to adequately accommodate issues central to adolescence such as cognitive and emotional developmental processes, issues of culture and ethnicity, the process of identity formation, the differential influence of environmental factors on adolescents' behaviour.

I returned to the literature in order to find some hints as to how to proceed, scanning the 'conclusion' sections for any discussions of the shortcomings of available theoretical frameworks. I wanted to know what accounts for the wide prevalence in adolescence of behaviours that are known to be unhealthy, known to elicit possible negative sanctions from society, criticism from parents or friends, and even self-rejection. How can we explain the lack of effectiveness of many of our health education efforts? What are the determinants of healthy behaviours in adolescence? As I reread, a recurring theme emerged that seemed essential. This theme suggested that adolescents tend to imbue behaviours with special, personal meanings, and that these meanings might be directly related to behaviour (Jessor, 1984; Perry, & Kelder, 1992). In Jessor's seminal chapter written in 1984, he suggested that important personal meanings of behaviour might play a central role in determining adolescent risk behaviour. He termed this the symbolic significance of behaviour or the psychological function of behaviour. He posited that risk behaviour is purposeful, goal-directed, and capable of fulfilling multiple goals that are central to adolescent life through the personal meanings with which adolescents imbue behaviours. These meanings are not intrinsic to the behaviour itself, but depend on larger processes of socio-cultural definition and the unique learning and socialisation experiences of an adolescent. Jessor generated a list of meanings or functions of adolescent risk behaviour to illustrate the point (Table 3.3).

These personal meanings of behaviour differ from expected outcomes, perceived benefits, or any of the comparable outcome constructs introduced in the value-expectancy theories. The strict multiplicative, linear, cause and effect temporal relationship between behaviour and outcome does not adequately represent the relationships between knowledge, events, emotions, motivations, and behaviour reflected in the personal meanings with which adolescents imbue behaviours. Personal meanings may not be related to external events, and they are often disassociated from available knowledge and information. Personal meanings of behaviour represent psychological functions of behaviour which are broader than outcome expectancies, although outcomes could conceivably be subsumed in the

TABLE 3.3

Jessor's list of personal meanings of behaviour

1. A way to attain goals that are blocked or seem otherwise unattainable (for instance, getting pregnant may represent gaining independence from parental control and take personal control of one's own life).

2. Rebellion against adult authority, norms and values of society.

3. A coping mechanism for dealing with anxiety, frustration, inadequacy, failure, fear of failure, anticipation of failure (school, expectations of peers or parents). Examples given here by Jessor are over eating, drug and alcohol abuse.

4. A way to gain admission/membership to peer group, expressing solidarity, demonstrate identification.

5. Confirmation of valued attributes of personal identity (macho, cool, experienced).

6. Transition marker, affirming maturity—indulging in age graded behaviours.

(Adapted from Jessor, 1984, pp.78–79)

construct. The meaning of binge eating, for instance, is related to the function of the activity, perhaps to ward off anxiety or to punish oneself, but also to the subjective symbolism of the food, perhaps as comfort, or an enemy, or something that must be internalised.

Several appeals had been made for more research into the personal, intrinsic meanings which adolescents often seem to attribute to health-related behaviour (Hurrelmann, 1990; Millstein, 1989; Perry, & Kelder, 1992). It seemed to me that the personal meanings of behaviour as defined here, purely intrinsic and emanating from personal feelings and fantasies, could be more influential for behaviour than any extrinsic incentive. Personal meanings of behaviour offered a single construct that might be researched independently or in conjunction with an extant theory. These meanings might be suited for applied research and field work, they could be used to direct intervention strategies and formulate programme goals. If this was the case, all the criteria for a 'good theory' could be met. At the outset, it was not my intention to formulate a new theory, in the light of the multitude of extant theories. But studying personal meanings of behaviour seemed the best path to take. In order to understand the content, form, and influence of these salient meanings of behaviour, I needed to go directly to the source. Much had been said about adolescents. I wanted to know how they felt about it themselves. Were there salient meanings that differentially guided their behaviours, and if so, what were these meanings? To proceed from the bottom up, as it were, demanded that I begin with qualitative research methods, to let the subjects speak.

PART TWO

Descriptive studies:
Letting the subjects speak

CHAPTER FOUR

Letting the subjects speak.
Part I: Taking inventory

INTRODUCTION

Phase one of the research was now complete. The major domains had been defined (Chapter 1), ethical issues had been reviewed and were in place (Chapter 2), and available theories had been explored (Chapter 3). To develop the second phase of the research, the results of the first phase had to be inventoried and then linked back to the original objective of the research, which was to develop and evaluate relevant and effective health education materials for adolescents concerning everyday health-related behaviours (see the Introduction). The information that had been accrued would guide further insights and decisions. So what was needed, what was known, and what were the lacunae in between?

To develop a *relevant* health education programme, the adolescents themselves must consider the material important and relevant for their own health. So information was needed on which areas of health Dutch adolescents found meaningful, on the structure and content of their knowledge in those areas, and on the nature of their most common health complaints. Moreover the material needs to be relevant to actual behaviour. Thus, information was needed on the everyday health-related behaviours of the target group. An *effective* health education programme was defined in this context as a programme that not only augments knowledge, but one that truly leads to behavioural change, and one which allows for the systematic evaluation of the individual contributions of each of the various components of the programme. To accomplish this, it is essential to know *why* the target group might engage in certain behaviours and shun others. In other words, to create effective health education, something must be known about the determinants of the behaviours to be addressed in the target group. We needed a viable theory of health-related behaviour.

A rich literature was emerging on adolescent risk behaviours such as tobacco use, drug abuse, alcohol abuse, and unsafe sexual practices. Less was available on health-related behaviour. Little data were available on the target group's knowledge concerning everyday health-related behaviours or their actual behaviour patterns, because the main focus in health education had been on risky behaviours (Van Asselt, & Lanphen, 1990; Donovan, Jessor, & Costa, 1991; Spruijt-Metz, & Spruijt, 1996). Little was known about Dutch adolescents' common health complaints, because this group ordinarily has a very low frequency of doctors' visits (with the exception of the chronically ill) (Lamberts, 1991). Finally, none of the existing theories seemed to adequately describe health-related behaviours in the target group. Moreover, most of the theories had been developed using samples of American white middle class college students (Sears, 1986). This contributed to conceptual bias, a lack of cultural sensitivity, and many pitfalls in the unadulterated application of these theories to other cultural groups within the United States (Graham, 1992; McLoyd, 1998). Even if the existing theories had been able to offer good descriptions of adolescent health behaviour within American samples, the direct workability of these theories in the Dutch culture would have been dubious.

Furthermore, The Netherlands' adolescent population is culturally extremely diverse and encompasses especially large Turkish, Moroccan, and Surinamese communities. This needed to be taken into account. Cultural diversity has repeatedly been related to differences in health status (Mackenbach, 1992; Netherlands Central Bureau of Statistics, 1992), health-related knowledge (Wilson et al., 1997b), and health behaviour (Organista et al., 1998; Wilson et al., 1997a). Different cultures may conceptualise sickness and health differently, value health differently, and uphold different health-related habits (Lewis, Belgrave, & Scott, 1990). Members of cultural minorities often belong to the lower socio-economic groups (Netherlands Central Bureau of Statistics, 1992). Low socio-economic status and poverty negatively influence health behaviour and health outcomes, and this relationship is still poorly understood (Earls, 1993; Jackson, & Sellers, 1997; McLoyd, & Ceballo, 1998). The unequal distribution of health among the economic groups in Holland despite the equal distribution of health care has been well documented (Mackenbach, 1992; Tax et al., 1984). However, little was available in the international literature about the differential effects of culture on adolescent health, health-related knowledge, health perceptions, or health behaviour. Next to nothing was available along these lines on the specific cultural groups in The Netherlands. At the beginning of this second phase, the research objective of developing and evaluating relevant and effective health education materials held for all Dutch adolescents, regardless of their cultural background. Information was therefore needed on health-related knowledge, health complaints, healthy and risky behaviour, and determinants of that behaviour from these different cultural groups.

After taking stock of these lacunae, five goals were set for the second phase of the research. These were: (1) to appraise current knowledge about health in the Dutch adolescent population, (2) to inventory perceived health and take stock of the health complaints of the group, (3) to assess health and risk behaviours adolescents undertake, (4) to explore the feasibility of reaching different cultural groups with the same material, and (5) to uncover possible determinants of health and risk behaviour. While no specific mention of gender differences is made in these goals, the study of gender differences is pertinent to most of them. Gender differences in perceived health, health complaints, and health behaviour have been noted by several authors (Cohen, Brownell, & Felix, 1990; Pennebaker, 1982; Spruijt-Metz, & Spruijt, 1996, 1997). We know that creating gender-specific interventions in adolescent health education can enhance effectiveness when indicated by preliminary research and when the differences are well understood (Flynn, Worden, Secker-Walker, Badger, & Geller, 1995). A preliminary examination of gender differences in health and health behaviour in the Dutch adolescent population was therefore included in this phase of the research.

Considering the magnitude of the above-mentioned lacunae, it was not possible to proceed directly to programme development, and extremely ill advised to proceed with any of the various forms of quantitative research. I wanted to talk directly to the adolescents, and was very curious about the ideas I had been developing from the first phase concerning the meanings of behaviour. The choice was made to make the second phase of research a qualitative one. I chose two related qualitative research techniques: a mainly open-ended questionnaire and a round of focus group interviews. This chapter reports on the questionnaire.

Box 4.1: What is qualitative research?

What is qualitative research? This is not an easy question to answer, because qualitative research is defined differently by different schools of researchers. The discussion has been animated and in some cases heated, and in the final analysis there is still little agreement. In Table 4.1 I have attempted to sort the different kinds of research that could be termed 'qualitative' into two schools, depending upon how the data are approached. In the accompanying text I will briefly try to sort out the agreements and disagreements among the different schools of qualitative researchers.

Table 4.1. Two groupings of 'Qualitative' research

	Research methods	Data	Data analysis techniques
School 1	Questionnaires, medical dossiers, but can also be used on data 'made' from interviews, visual or observational data, field notes	Categorical data (nominal or ordinal level) gathered or 'made'	Non-parametric (tests) various model types for categorical data such as loglinear and logit, optimal scaling techniques
School 2	Interviews, observation, field notes, videos, texts	Text and visual materials	Coding, clustering, contrasting, comparing

Box 4.1 continued

Box 4.1: What is qualitative research? (continued)

School 1 is represented by statisticians such as Alan Agresti (Agresti, 1990). This school holds that categorical variables (measured at the nominal or ordinal level) are "qualitative—distinct levels differ in quality, not in quantity" (Agresti, 1990, p. 4). Categorical variables use measuring scales that are made up of categories, like religious affiliation (Catholic, Jewish, Protestant, Islamic, other). Religious affiliation is an example of a nominal variable, because it does not have ordered levels. Ordinal variables do have ordered levels, like social class (upper, middle, lower). Researchers from this school use non-parametric techniques to analyse their data. These techniques range from simple frequency tables and chi square tests through the various types of models for categorical data, such at loglinear models, logit models, and optimal scaling techniques. This school of research considers counting responses and testing hypotheses indispensable aspects of data analysis.

School 2 is represented by ethnographic researchers such as Denzin and Lincoln (1994) and Miles and Huberman (1994). Here are some points of agreement among the various factions in this school:

◆ Qualitative data consists of text rather than numbers.

◆ Qualitative research is usually conducted using an intense or prolonged contact with a 'field' or 'life' situation.

◆ The situations studied are usually 'naturalistic'.

◆ Every effort is made to get an overview of the context in which the subjects function.

◆ To various conceptual degrees, qualitative researchers emphasise getting to know the 'other', capturing data on the perceptions of the subjects 'from the inside'.

◆ An important aim of the research is to understand how people in their own settings come to understand, explain, behave.

◆ Little standard instrumentation is used, especially in early phases of research.

Within this second school, the disagreement about how to analyse the data persists. Some consider counting responses and other 'quantitatively related' practices to be useful components of the analytical arsenal (Krippendorff, 1980), and will 'borrow' from quantitative techniques if it suits their needs. Others feel very strongly that reducing text to numbers is anathema for the qualitative tradition and should be reserved for quantitative methods (Silverman, 1993). How one envisions the process of data analysis has far-reaching consequences for all steps of the research as well as for the epistemological point of departure. This debate still rages.

I am a quantitatively trained researcher who came to qualitative research techniques and data analysis because I felt that I could not accomplish my research agenda using solely quantitative methods. I try to move between the schools depending upon which suits the research at the moment. In my opinion, qualitative and quantitative methods are complementary, equally valuable, and best used together at different junctions in the process of research, depending upon the knowledge available and the questions at hand.

Box 4.2: When are qualitative research techniques indicated?

Making distinctions on when one would use the different qualitative research techniques is perhaps the best way to discriminate between the two schools outlined in Box 4.1. De Groot (1961) maintained that empirical research proceeded in five stages, which he called the empirical cycle (Table 4.2).

Table 4.2. de Groot's empirical cycle

Stage	Activities
1. Observation (in the general sense of observing *reality*, rather than of observing *subjects*, which comes later	➤ Literature study ➤ Collection and grouping of empirical fact material ➤ Forming theories
2. Induction	➤ Formulating general hypotheses ➤ Formalisation of theory ➤ From specific observations in stage one to general hypotheses ➤ Choosing constructs
3. Deduction	➤ From general hypotheses to specific concrete, testable prediction ➤ Filling in constructs and predicting relationships between constructs
4. Testing	➤ The business of experimental, quasi-experimental, and descriptive studies ➤ Operationalisation of constructs ➤ Measurement ➤ Look for correlation between variables
5. Evaluation	➤ Establish worth, meaning of results in wider context, in context of theory from stage one, general hypotheses from stage 2, and specific predictions from stage 3. How do they interrelate? ➤ Do results support? Falsify? How strong is the evidence? ➤ Are the results generalisable? ➤ What are the practical implications? ➤ Is there new input? Does it warrant changes in theory? Back to stage 1!

The qualitative research techniques from School 1 are useful when constructs are most accurately operationalised using categorical variables. These techniques allow us to build models and test hypotheses using non-numerical data. These techniques lend themselves most to the fourth and fifth stages of the empirical cycle. They are usually used when research questions have been framed,

Box 4.2 continued

Box 4.2: When are qualitative research techniques indicated? (continued)

constructs have been operationalised, and hypotheses are to some extent in place. In terms of de Groot's empirical cycle, these techniques are most useful in the fourth and fifth stages.

The qualitative research techniques from School 2 are more suited to the first three stages of the empirical cycle. These techniques are ideal for generating theory, identifying important constructs, and filling in these constructs conceptually. In my research, I used interview techniques to see if my theoretical ideas had any resonance within the target group. Qualitative research methods from School 2 can help to pinpoint and flesh out the constructs relevant to the research in the population of interest. For instance, in developing smoking prevention programmes for adolescents, Worden et al.'s group (1988) conducted a preliminary round of focus group interviews to explore young people's needs for smoking prevention, their interests, and their lifestyles. Qualitative research techniques from School 2 can be used to determine the breadth of a construct within and across populations (Knight, & Hill, 1998). They are thus extremely useful in cross-cultural research. They can be used very effectively to identify variables and frame hypotheses for quantitative research, bridging the gap between stages three and four of De Groot's empirical cycle (Weiss, 1994). Above and beyond these advantages, qualitative research methods from the second school offer an excellent opportunity to get to know your target group (Jessor, Colby, & Shewder, 1996).

Addressing the five goals

The first goal of this round—appraising health-related knowledge—was left entirely for the interview. Since specific realms of behaviour addressed in the later phases of research and development were to be chosen according to the information from this phase, I would not yet have known what questions to ask. To cover the second goal—taking inventory of common health complaints—existing questionnaires were translated and pilot tested. The third goal—assessing health and risk behaviours—was addressed with open questions about behaviour. The fourth goal—having to do with possible cultural differences—was addressed by drawing a multi-cultural sample for this phase of the research.

The fifth goal, the study of determinants of health-related behaviour, remained central in this second phase of the research. No adequate theory of adolescent health-related behaviour had emerged from the first phase of the research, and I was not far enough along in my conceptualisation of the meanings of behaviour to use written measures or open questions. However, several more descriptive constructs from the literature showed promise as possible determinants of everyday health-related behaviour in adolescents. It made sense to pilot-test these constructs for their possible predictive value in a small sample. This study focused on four potential determinants of health and risk behaviour: psychological well-being, affectivity, family communications, and religious affiliation. Here is the rationale for these choices.

Research had shown that psychological well-being as expressed by measures such as stress, loneliness and daily hassles has a great impact on adolescent health (Hurrelmann, 1990). In an attempt to further specify the nature of that impact, this preliminary research explored the relationships between psychological well-being, symptom reporting, health and risk behaviours.

Watson and Pennebaker (1989) partition affectivity into two distinct concepts: positive affectivity and negative affectivity. Positive affectivity represents good mood and high energy, while negative affectivity represents a general dimension of subjective distress. Watson and Pennebaker found that high levels of health complaints were related to negative affectivity, while positive affectivity was unrelated to any of several scales for physical complaints. In this study, I chose to explore connections between negative affectivity and experiencing more symptoms among Dutch adolescents, and to investigate possible links between the initiation of health or risk behaviours and positive or negative affectivity.

The relationship between family tensions and psychosomatic disorders in adolescence has been discussed repeatedly in the literature (Hurrelmann, Engel, Holler, & Nordlohne, 1988; Resnick et al., 1997). Interpersonal communication skills have also been identified as central to preventive health education (Swisher, 1976). Here the relationship between symptom reporting, health behaviours, risk behaviours and the quality of family communications was examined.

Interest in the buffering effects of religious affiliation against adolescents' involvement in risk behaviour has grown exponentially in the United States since its inclusion in Jessor's Problem Behaviour theory (Jessor, 1984). Religious affiliation has successfully predicted the performance of fewer risk behaviours among American youths in several studies (Benson, & Donahue, 1989; Jessor, 1984). It was decided to explore the value of this predictor among the Dutch youth.

METHODS

There are several advantages to using a small-scale qualitative type questionnaire in conjunction with interviews. Gathering questionnaire-type data alongside interview data provides convergent operationalisations of important constructs (Cook, & Campbell, 1979). In this research, the open-ended part of the questionnaire allowed the adolescents themselves to generate relevant items for later, quantitative phases of the research. Allowing the target group to generate their own questionnaires proved to be a great asset in the later phases of the research. Another major advantage of using this convergent design was that extant questionnaires could be pilot tested for their usefulness and relevance within this particular group of adolescents. After responding to the questionnaires, we discussed their reactions in the group. This was especially useful for questionnaires translated from other languages or meant for other samples. Pilot testing also provides the opportunity to check the validity and reliability of wording and scaling of single items before using them in a large-scale quantitative study. In an interview situation, it can happen that some of the topics on the agenda get skipped if other topics take off or new subjects come to the fore. Using a questionnaire to complement the interview protocol ensures that the topics on the questionnaire would be covered in every group. Finally, in a group interview situation, not every participant will contribute to the discussion of all topics equally. Using the questionnaire in conjunction with the interviews ensured that responses from all group participants were available for each topic on the questionnaire.

Subjects

Fifty-three adolescents between the ages of 12 and 16 participated in this project: 36 Dutch adolescents and 17 adolescents with Turkish or Moroccan backgrounds. The 36 Dutch adolescents came from one large school community including college preparatory as well as regular high-school classes. They were asked to participate in the study during school hours. The parents received written information on the project and gave formal permission. An equal number of boys and girls evenly covering the range of ages between 12 and 16 were selected.

The 17 Turkish and Moroccan adolescents were either born in Turkey or Morocco, or first generation Dutch (both parents being immigrants). They were recruited from homework help programmes in two community centres. These two cultural groups were placed together in this study because they occurred so in the ad hoc sampling. Turkish and Moroccan people living in The Netherlands often share the same neighbourhoods. They share the heritage of Islam, and their socio-economic status is comparable. For these reasons, and considering the small sample size it was considered feasible to combine the two groups for this study. The participants were asked by the teachers to participate in their free time and received gift certificates for participation.

Procedure

For the questionnaire/interview phase, the main researcher and an observer were present at all times. We met with small groups of participants (5 to 7 in each group) in a room provided by the school, and at the two community centres. After a brief introduction to the research, the adolescents filled in the questionnaire individually and subsequently took part in the focus group interview. The questionnaire took about 30 minutes to complete. The open-ended questions required some thought.

Variables

General questions concerning demographic variables and religious affiliation were followed by a group of variables concerning psychological well-being affect, social network, symptoms, and health-related behaviours.

Psychological well-being. Perceived health was rated on a five-point scale, tiredness in the morning and loneliness were rated on four-point scales. A 12 item 'worry list' made up of statements such as "I worry about the way I look", compiled from preliminary interviews and other existing questionnaires, was filled in (Van Asselt, & Lanphen, 1990). The adolescents were asked to choose up to three relevant worries. There was also space provided to fill in their own most pressing worry or concern. For the quantitative analyses, the number of times that the various worries were chosen was counted.

The affectivity scale. Negative or positive affectivity was assessed with a three-item scale (Cronbach's alpha .78) including frequency of bad moods, feeling lousy, and being nervous. The items were scored from 1 (never) to 5 (often). The scale was distilled from Watson and Pennebaker's work (1989).

Social network. Communication with the parents was scored on a four-point scale where the subjects rate how easy (or difficult) it is to communicate with each parent about things that are bothering them.

Symptom report. The Dutch version of the Pennebaker Inventory for Limbic Languidness (PILL) was included in the questionnaire (Cronbach's alpha .92) (Pennebaker, 1982; Spruijt & Spruijt-Metz, 1994; Van Vliet, 1992). The respondents rated the frequency with which they were bothered by each of 52 symptoms on a five-point scale. This questionnaire was designed to measure the tendency to report symptoms. Here, the PILL was also used to rank the symptoms according to prevalence among the adolescents. To check the understanding of (semi-) medical vocabulary, the participants were requested to underline any word that they did not understand. After underlining words they did not understand, help was available from the researchers for filling in the PILL. The mean score of the items they understood (including those that required help) was used in the analyses.

Health and risk behaviours. Health behaviours and risk behaviours undertaken were inventoried by asking the adolescents to describe in their own words what they did to stay healthy and what they did that they knew may be harmful for their health. They could name as many health or risk behaviours undertaken that they could think of. For the quantitative analyses, the number of health behaviours and risk behaviours mentioned was counted.

Statistical analyses: Proceed with caution

Before we look at results from this preliminary questionnaire, it must be remarked that this was an exploratory phase of research. The small sample size meant that the power of the tests was very low, so we need to be very circumspect when we talk about significance in the statistical sense (Cohen, 1988). Why bother to do the analyses, might then be the question? This kind of preliminary data can give great insight into what works and what does not work within a population. The information from the statistical 'tests' gave extra input that was collated with the information gathered from the interview data and observations. These preliminary analyses (sometimes called 'snooping the data') contributed to the building of a more valid questionnaire for the later large-scale survey by guiding decisions about the inclusion and exclusion of items and variables (results are reported in Chapters 6, 7, and 8). These analyses were hypothesis generating rather than hypothesis testing. They were used to help provide answers to questions that would guide further research questions (such as which constructs should be included?) and further research design (such as which populations and what kind of manipulations should be included?).

RESULTS

Table 4.3 shows the ten highest scored symptoms on the PILL, the health and risk behaviours mentioned in order of frequency, and the 10 most frequently chosen worries from the worry list in descending order of frequency.

The worry most frequently added to the worry list in the space provided was 'worries about love'. The scores on the PILL showed that headaches are frequent, with 78% of the sample reporting occasional to frequent headaches. Most of the Dutch subjects understood all the items, and did not underline any of them. The Turkish/Moroccan adolescents generally underlined between one-third and one-half of the list, so the medical vocabulary seemed to differ between the two groups. The PILL could therefore not be used for both in a survey situation.

TABLE 4.3

Symptoms, health behaviours, risk behaviours, and worries in descending order of importance

Top ten symptoms in descending order of intensity	Health behaviours in descending order of frequency	Risk behaviours in descending order of frequency	Worries in descending order of frequency
Acne	Sport	Not enough sport	The future
Headache	Healthy eating habits	Unhealthy eating habits	Appearance
Stuffy nose	Enough sleep	Not enough sleep	Feelings in a knot
Blushing	Warm clothing	No warm clothing	Being bored
Coughing	Vitamins	Smoking/drinking	Grades
Sneezing	Hygiene	Walkman too loud	Achievements of goals
Runny nose	Not smoking/drinking		Problems with parents
Oversensitive teeth	Hobbies		Wish I were different
Back pain	Having fun		Problems with friends
Sore throat	Dental hygiene		Being alone
			Money
			Health

Box 4.3: Finding your way through the statistics in 'Result' sections

For some of the readers of this book, statistics might be very intimidating and inaccessible. For other readers, however, results would be considered incomplete and difficult to interpret if they are presented verbally without the statistics. Indeed, statistics are an essential part of scientific argumentation. We use statistics to demonstrate how we came to our conclusions and to allow other scientists to check our conclusions and form their own opinions. I have chosen to leave the statistics in the text, because I feel that it is richer and more informative if they are included. I hope the following remarks on reading statistics will be helpful for readers who might feel less comfortable with them.

◆ **Reading it all?**

In the first place, keep in mind that even scientists who are perfectly at home with statistical techniques do not customarily work through all the statistics in a result section in detail. They will most likely scan over the statistics and only delve deeply into a particular result that interests them, or into an unfamiliar statistical technique that might be of use to them, or into a result that appears irregular in order to check it. So 'reading' a result section does not necessarily mean going over every table in detail.

◆ **Tables and figures**

Aside from the tables, which portray the statistics in numbers, there are also figures in most of the ensuing results sections. These represent the statistics graphically and are often easier to understand than the tables. The figures frequently portray the various group averages, which facilitates comparisons. If you begin with reading the texts and glancing at the figures, you can always decide that a particular table is of interest and go back to study it. An excellent companion book is *Using Multivariate Statistics* (Tabachnick, & Fidell, 1996).

◆ **Skipping the 'Results' sections**

All the chapters that include statistics (Chapters 4, 6, 7, 8, and 9) end with a Discussion section. The discussion section always includes an interpretation of the statistical results. Some people skip the Results sections entirely and go directly from the Methods section to the Discussion section. While this approach is not uncommon, it severely limits your perspective. It does offer an interpretation of the statistical results, but it will not enable you to trace the origins of the interpretation or conclusions. Statistics are the epistemological anchor of empirical research. Statistics are the evidence of the empirical grounding of research in experience and observations. If you skip them entirely, it will be difficult to form an opinion on the validity of the research.

◆ **A perspective on multivariate statistical techniques**

Finally, the book as a whole covers a fairly broad spectrum of multivariate statistics, each of them put into their particular place in the larger project. Fairly detailed descriptions of why particular tests are suitable for particular data, of how to deal with messy data and of the strengths and weaknesses of particular analysis techniques are regularly included. Hopefully, the result sections taken together will convey an idea of the various types of available techniques and how to fit them to different kinds of data and research questions.

Gender and cultural differences on symptom report, health behaviour, and risk behaviour

ANOVAs (analyses of variance) were used instead of t-tests because they also test for interactions between gender and ethnicity, which would not be possible using a series of t-tests. ANOVAs were also preferable because this technique makes multiple comparisons using only one test. Due to the small sample size, it was important to get as much information as possible using as few tests as possible.

In an analysis of variance on the PILL scores, a trend for an interaction effect between gender and cultural group was found ($F = 3.83$, df = 1, 48, $p = .056$). Figure 4.1 shows this trend.

A significant difference was found on PILL scores between Dutch boys and Dutch girls ($t = -2.25$, df = 33, $p = .03$) and between Dutch girls and Turkish / Moroccan girls ($t = 2.19$, df = 25, $p = .04$).

Dutch girls reported more symptoms than Dutch boys. This is in keeping with the vast literature on symptom reporting in Western societies, which shows that females of all ages report more physical symptoms than their male counterparts (Bush, Harkings, Harrington, & Price, 1993; Donovan, Jessor, & Costa, 1993; Kaufman, Brown, Graves, Henderson, & Revolinski, 1993; McGuire, Mitic, & Neumann, 1987; Pennebaker, 1982; Spruijt-Metz, & Spruijt, 1996). Figure 4.1 suggests that the roles seemed to be reversed in the Turkish–Moroccan groups. In this subsample, the boys tended to report more symptoms than the girls.

Analyses of variance on health and risk behaviours were conducted to see if there were any differences in behaviours between the genders or ethnic groups. Results from these analyses are presented in Tables 4.4a and 4.4b,

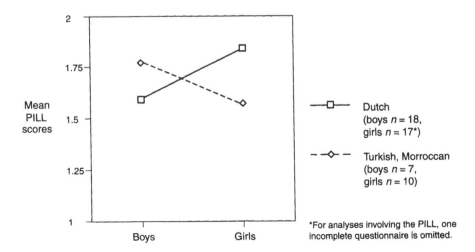

FIG. 4.1   Interaction between gender and ethnic group on PILL scores.

TABLE 4.4a

Analyses of variance on effects of gender and ethnicity
on health behaviours

Variable	Health behaviours undertaken		
	F	df	p
Gender	.23	1, 49	.63
Ethnicity	4.95	1, 49	.03*
Sex * Ethnicity	.17	1, 49	.69

TABLE 4.4b

Analyses of variance on effects of gender and ethnicity
on risk behaviours

Variable	Health behaviours undertaken		
	F	df	p
Gender	4.18	1, 49	.05*
Ethnicity	7.80	1, 49	.01*
Sex * Ethnicity	.09	1, 49	.77

No interactions were found. There was a main effect of ethnicity on health
behaviour, as shown in Fig. 4.4a. The Dutch youth report more health behaviour
than the Turkish and Moroccan youths.

For risk behaviour, main effects were found for both gender and ethnicity. Dutch
adolescents report more risk behaviour than Turkish or Moroccan adolescents, and
girls report more risk behaviour than boys. Figure 4.3 offers a graphic representation
of the cell means.

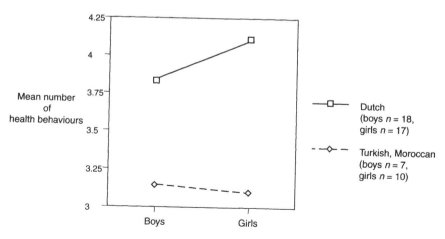

FIG. 4.2   Mean number of health behaviours reported.

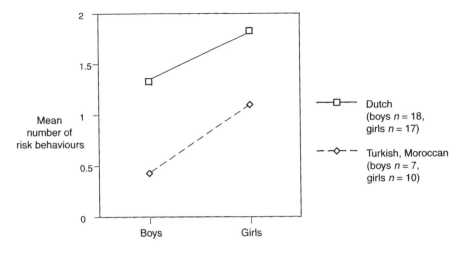

FIG. 4.3   Mean number of risk behaviours reported.

Psychological well-being

Cronbach's alpha for the variables representing psychological well-being was low (.43), suggesting that the variables may represent different aspects of psychological well-being. Therefore, individual items were used for the analyses instead of forcing these items into one 'scale'.

No gender or ethnic differences were found in perceived health or tiredness. The Dutch adolescents scored lower on loneliness ($F = 1.82$, df = 1, 48, $p = 0.40$) than the Turkish/Moroccan adolescents. An interaction was found between gender and ethnicity on loneliness ($F = 4.83$, df = 1, 48, $p = .03$). Girls in both ethnic groups reported about the same levels of loneliness, while the Turkish/Moroccan boys scored considerably higher than both groups of girls and the Dutch boys. Girls reported consistently more worries than boys ($F = 5.94$, df = 1, 49, $p = .02$).

The correlations between the psychological well-being variables and symptom reporting, health behaviour, and risk behaviour are shown in Table 4.5. While loneliness and tiredness correlate with the PILL, worries and perceived health do not.

TABLE 4.5

Correlations between the psychological well-being variables and PILL scores, health behaviours, and risk behaviours

	Perceived health	*Tiredness*	*Loneliness*	*Worries*
PILL	.24	.40**	.37**	.17
Health behaviours	.03	-.06	-.10	-.09
Risk behaviours	.15	.11	.06	.04

**p<.01

The affectivity scale

No effects for gender or ethnic group were found on the affectivity scale. The scale correlated significantly with PILL scores ($r = .56, p = .01$), and with risk behaviour ($r = .36, p = .01$). No relationship was found with health behaviours.

Ease of communications

No effects for ethnicity were found in ease of communications. Gender differences were found in both communications with the mother ($F = 6.97$, df = 1, 47, $p = .01$) and with father ($F = 3.89$, df = 1,40, $p = .056$). In both cases, the girls report more difficulty in communications with the parents. Only communication with the father correlated negatively with PILL scores ($r = -.30, p = .05$): better communications with the father is related to fewer reported symptoms.

Stepwise multiple regression analyses on the PILL scores, health and risk behaviour

For the regression analyses, the following variables were entered after snooping the data for the variables with the most predictive value: the affectivity scale, the psychological well-being items, and the communication with father. Table 4.6 shows the results of the stepwise regression analysis on the PILL scores.

For health behaviour, none of the variables significantly contributed to the regression equation. For risk behaviour, some variance was explained by the affectivity scale ($R^2 = .10$, Beta = .31).

A final round of regression analyses was performed adding the PILL scores to the equation for both health and risk behaviours. Although the PILL correlated with risk behaviour ($r = .29, p = .05$), symptom report as operationalised by the PILL did not explain any variance for either health or risk behaviour.

Religious affiliation was evenly distributed over the different cultural groups and over the genders. No relationship between religious affiliation and number of health or risk behaviours undertaken was found.

DISCUSSION

A tired, lonely adolescent reports more symptoms and is moody. An adolescent who reports more symptoms and is moody will engage in more risk behaviour.

TABLE 4.6

Stepwise multiple regression on PILL scores

Step	Variable	Beta	R^2	R^2 change
1	Affectivity scale	.59	.34	–
2	Loneliness	.36	.46	.12

This is the picture that emerges from the data. The finding on the relationship between communications with the father and symptom report is curious, and perhaps replication should precede interpretation.

Considering the small sample size, the effects found were numerous and large. This will partially be due to the variance introduced by the cognitive and socio-economic differences between the ethnic groups. The Dutch high-school students in the sample attend a high school in a good neighbourhood that prepares them for white-collar jobs, college and university. Most of the Turkish/Moroccan students in the sample attend high schools in a lower class neighbourhood, which prepare them for trade and trade schools. This may mean that the differences found are representative, but are perhaps amplified by the sample selection. It may also mean that these differences are not simply attributable to ethnicity, but also have to do with lower levels of SES and cognitive development, which are in turn often part and parcel of minority status.

Having said this, the analyses involving health and risk behaviours and PILL scores point to major differences between the Dutch group and the Turkish/Moroccan group. That females report more and more intense symptoms has been well documented in Western cultures (Bush et al., 1993; Newcomb, & Bentler, 1987; Spruijt, & Spruijt-Metz, 1994; Spruijt-Metz, & Spruijt, 1996). In this sample, the Dutch adolescents adhere to these earlier results while the reverse is found in the Turkish/Moroccan group. The differences in number of health and risk behaviours reported could reflect different life-styles, which again may implicate differences in SES, confounded by ethnic differences. These findings indicated that reaching such different ethnic groups with the same lesson materials might not succeed. Supplementary materials backed by substantial knowledge of these cultures and taking their specific needs into consideration would need to be made.

Gender differences were found on symptom reporting, risk behaviours, worries, and ease of communication with parents. In the literature, gender differences have been found in other areas such as anxiety and depression (Avison, & Mcalpine, 1992; Gore, Aseltine, & Colton, 1992). This suggests that differences in the affectivity scale and some of the psychological well-being variables might have been found in a larger sample. The question arose, should the same conclusion be drawn with respect to the genders as with respect to the cultures. Because the shared culture affords an underlying network of shared concepts, and because these concepts are also shared by the researchers involved in making the lesson materials, we chose not to make materials for boys and girls separately. However, these gender differences may not be ignored. Perry and Kelder (1992) offer several suggestions for the involvement of the peer group in the health education process, and Hølund (1990) shows that peer-group teachers change their own behaviours by teaching healthy habits to others. Recent evidence has shown that peer-group teachers can boost the efficacy of prevention efforts in heterogeneous groups (Huba, & Melchior, 1998; Sloboda,

& David, 1997). Strategic planning of peer group teaching offers one option for taking gender differences into account. For instance, a number of separate sessions on the same materials could be led by girls for all-girl groups and by boys for all-boy groups. Discussions of risky and healthy behaviours and their ramifications could be placed in the context of gender-specific motivations and needs. This should be augmented by further research into possible gender-specific determinants of health and risk behaviour.

It is almost impossible to differentiate between symptom perception and symptom report, and we can only rarely differentiate between symptom report and physical phenomena: we usually cannot verify a stomach ache (Spruijt, & Hoogstraten, 1992). We are frequently forced to accept symptom reporting as our best representation of symptom perception, and often our only representation of physical symptoms. Keeping this in mind, the fact that 78% of the sample report occasional to frequent headache indicates that lesson material on causes and prevention of this and several of the other highest scoring complaints would be relevant. Elements such as mood and loneliness were shown to play an important role in the reporting of symptoms. The questions arise: to what extent do they contribute to the actual perception of symptoms, or to the actual prevalence of symptoms? For our purposes, these findings point to the imperative of teaching mental health skills along with physical health skills.

None of the variables contributed to the prediction of the frequency with which health behaviours were undertaken, and only negative affectivity contributed a bit to the prediction of risk behaviour. It is important to note that none of these basic experiences: being lonely, tired, moody, worried, or experiencing more symptoms, show a relationship with taking positive action in the form of health behaviour, such as getting more sleep or talking about problems. Perhaps this is due to the low priority of health and the little thought that health is accorded. Health did not figure highly on the worry list. The adolescents in this sample are not particularly concerned about their health; it is not something that they think about much. There are several indications that logical connections between perceived well-being and personal behaviour are not being made. For instance, although 'feelings in a knot' scored number three on the worry list, no mention of talking about problems or dealing with feelings was made on the health behaviour list.

Evidence that logical connections are not being made was also found in the comments frequently added to the answers on the open questions. For instance, descriptions spontaneously offered for 'healthy eating habits' as a healthy behaviour often showed a lack of understanding as to what this means. While healthy eating habits are part of the school curriculum, 'healthy eating habits' when applied to personal behaviour seems to be, in some cases, a much heard, empty slogan, as do a number of other expressions, such as 'sport and exercise'. Also, the same person who reports 'healthy eating habits' as a health behaviour may just as well report 'eating lots of candy and chips' as a risk behaviour frequently undertaken.

Furthermore, the participants came up with relatively few risk behaviours. This suggests that some common behaviours in this sample such as bicycling through a red light, are not consciously connected to health risk.

The lack of results concerning religious affiliation indicates that the effect of religion on health and risk behaviour found by several American researchers might either be culture or religion specific. Replication with larger samples in several other countries differentiating for type of religion might yield some interesting results.

Going back to the five goals of this study: (1) the assessment of health and risk behaviours offers a sound basis for further research. The focus group interviews in the next phase of this study will concentrate on how well the adolescents understand the health and risk behaviours they report, and which determinants they give for their behaviour. (2) The current knowledge about health (and health-risk) may be at least partly comprised of empty slogans and what might be termed 'free floating facts': facts that are not embedded in a relevant context of cause and effect. Here again, results from focus group interviews may offer some clarity by examining the health-related knowledge in depth. (3) The health inventories point towards some topics that would be relevant for inclusion in health education materials, such as information on frequently occurring complaints like headache. Social skills and strategies for dealing with loneliness, mood swings, and worries are also candidates for inclusion. (4) On the strength of these preliminary findings, it was not deemed feasible to reach the different cultural groups involved in this research relying solely on the same lesson material. I was convinced that supplementary material addressing the specific needs and interests of the minority groups would be needed. To accomplish this and to do a good job of it, two possibilities were open. One was to hire new team-members that were knowledgeable about these ethnic groups or preferably members of these groups themselves. The other was to extend the project substantially in order to give me the time to delve into the rich and complex cultures of the main minority groups in The Netherlands. Since neither of these possibilities could be supported financially, the decision was made to proceed only for the Dutch adolescents, abandoning the research for the Turkish and Moroccan adolescents for the time being.

Lastly, let us turn to the fifth goal concerning determinants of health and risk behaviours. Psychological well-being, affectivity, communications with the parents, and religious affiliation did not function as determinants of behaviour in this sample. What motivates adolescents to undertake health behaviours if not factors related to physical, psychological, and social health as incorporated in this study? The material points to cognitive inconsistencies that may indicate that rational models are of questionable value in understanding why adolescents undertake health and risk behaviours. The personal meaning of behaviour, sometimes referred to as the psychological function of behaviour (Hurrelmann, 1990; Jessor, 1984; Perry, & Kelder, 1992) rose in my estimation as a possible determinant for health and risk behaviours in adolescence. We now turn to the analysis of the focus group interviews. In the interviews, the adolescents themselves are given a chance to speak about what various behaviours mean to them. The meanings that they ascribe to health-related behaviours are examined for their credibility as determinants of these behaviours.

CHAPTER FIVE

Letting the subjects speak.
Part II: The focus group interviews

INTRODUCTION

The idea that adolescents imbue behaviours with personal meanings and that these meanings then become important behavioural determinants is a compelling one. Meanings of behaviour have periodically been put forth as possible determinants of both health and risk behaviours in adolescence (Hurrelmann, 1990; Jessor, 1984; Perry, & Kelder, 1992; Tappe, 1992), but research on them has been minimal. To obtain a greater understanding of health and risk behaviours and their meanings for the target group, focus group interviews were chosen as the most appropriate method. The imperative of social diagnosis in the process of designing successful intervention programmes has been stressed (Green, & Kreuter, 1991). The importance of qualitative approaches for this purpose has accrued wide recognition (Creswell, 1998; Denzin, & Lincoln, 1994; Jessor, Colby, & Shewder, 1996; Khan et al., 1991; Krueger, 1994; Miles, & Huberman, 1994; Moore, 1987; Morgan, 1997; Silverman, 1993; Stewart, & Shamdasani, 1990; Weiss, 1994). However, some researchers have eloquently expressed their doubts concerning the adequacy of the exclusive use of quantitative approaches (Khan et al., 1991). Studies rarely bring together inventories of specific health behaviours, overviews of the prevalence of relevant knowledge and skills, and studies of motivations and determinants of behaviours for one group of adolescents (Cohen, Brownell, & Felix, 1990). However, information from all these areas need to be amalgamated to create a comprehensive body of knowledge upon which to base interventions. These were the considerations that prompted the combination of the preliminary questionnaire with interview techniques to bring together several areas of information in one study.

In the interviews, the participants were asked to elaborate upon their general knowledge, values, attitudes, beliefs and feelings concerning health to assure the development of relevant health education materials. The adolescents' understanding of specific health behaviours and risk behaviours within the predetermined domains of everyday health-related behaviour was investigated. To address the problem of creating effective materials, the meanings of health and risk behaviours were probed, and the function of the meaning of behaviour as a determinant of adolescent health and risk behaviours was examined.

METHODS

In focus group interviews, a moderator directs the discussion between six to twelve members of the target population according to a flexible protocol. This type of research offers a rapid assessment technique that has several advantages over other qualitative, in-depth techniques. It provides in-depth information without requiring full-scale anthropological investigations, and offers the opportunity to observe a large amount of interaction on a chosen topic in a limited period of time. While a variety of research needs lend themselves to the use of focus groups, they are especially useful for idea generation and hypothesis building (Morgan, 1997). Group interactions often stimulate memories and feelings, and promote brainstorming between group members. This affords the opportunity to explore the relevance of unexpected issues, which may crop up during brainstorming. The likelihood of participants generating answers because they think it might please the interviewer is reduced in a group of peers. Participants may feel more secure as it becomes evident that an idea or feeling can be exposed without necessarily being forced to defend statements, follow through or elaborate (Green, & Kreuter, 1991; Khan et al., 1991; Stewart, & Shamdasani, 1990).

While focus group interviews offer many research advantages, the limitations of focus groups must also be kept in mind. These are for the most part the same limitations that are associated with most qualitative research methodologies. The samples are small and purposefully selected, which does not allow for direct generalisation to larger populations. Responses may be influenced by the moderator and by the other participants. This forms a threat to the reliability and validity of the data. The chance of introducing bias and subjectivity into the interpretation of the data must not be underestimated (Green, & Kreuter, 1991; Khan et al., 1991; Stewart, & Shamdasani, 1990). It is particularly tempting to count people participating in focus group research rather than the number of groups. However, the responses from members of the group are not independent of one another. Therefore, the group is considered to be the fundamental unit of analysis in this study (Morgan, 1997; Stewart, & Shamdasani, 1990).

Sample and design

The same subjects that filled in the questionnaire described in Chapter 4 participated in the focus group interviews described here. The 36 Dutch adolescents were placed into six groups of six subjects. Three groups were made up of regular high school students, and the other three were made up of college preparatory students. For each high school type, one all-girl group, one all-boy group, and one mixed group were formed. These were carefully stratified so that the participants were not classmates, and there was an even distribution of ages (12–17 years old). The reason for this choice of grouping is that while some topics may lend themselves to discussion in mixed groups, other topics may be easier to address in homogeneous groups of boys or girls separately (Khan et al., 1991). The 17 Turkish and Moroccan adolescents were split into three groups: two all-girl groups (5 girls each) and one all-boy group (7 boys). Upon the advice of the teachers, no mixed groups were created. The main arguments against forming mixed groups concerned cultural taboos that rest upon the discussion of many of the topics in the interview protocol with members of the opposite sex.

Procedure

The adolescents filled in the questionnaire and subsequently took part in a focus group interview. The focus groups were made up of the five to seven participants, a moderator, and an observer. In the present research, the observer was a medical professional who did not participate actively in the interviews unless specific medical questions arose. Filling in the questionnaire took approximately 30 minutes, and the interview took approximately 90 minutes.

The focus group interviews reported here are semi-structured interviews, sometimes bordering on 'self managing groups' (Morgan, 1997). The protocol (Table 5.1) was established using material collected in several preliminary in-depth interviews with adolescents. The order of topics in the protocol was not strictly followed, and if relevant topics arose that were not included, the moderator could depart from the protocol at her discretion. While there were some initial doubts as to the length of the sitting (90 minutes), the subjects seemed interested and motivated, and often remained after the interview for informal discussion. The interviews were recorded on cassette tape with permission of the participants. Analyses were conducted using typed transcripts of the tapes.

ANALYSIS

A content analysis of the interviews was undertaken. First, thematic content units were defined. Thematic content units are interpretative or explanatory sets of statements on themes within the interview (Stewart, & Shamdasani, 1990). Thus, a thematic content unit is partially a product of the interview protocol itself because it informs the topics to be discussed, and partly a product of what the participants say because they fill in the recurring themes. Defining content units is an iterative process. Twenty-one thematic content units were found by bouncing back and forth

TABLE 5.1

Protocol for the interviews

Information given at school and at home concerning health and medicine
Information the adolescents feel that they need or would like to have
The subjective meaning and value of health
Specific health and risk behaviours undertaken
Perceived personal and parental responsibility for own health
Attitude towards general practitioner, frequency of and reasons for doctor's visit
Path to doctor: Who takes initiative, knowledge of health insurance, perceived availability of
    services
Types and frequencies of self-medication undertaken
Perception of physical changes and sexuality in puberty
Ease of, and need for communication about feelings
Breaking rules, 'sneaking,' authority, autonomy, and health and risk behaviours
'Magic wand' round: desired changes in self and surroundings

between the original protocol and the information found in the transcripts of the interviews (Table 5.2).

The interview transcripts were then coded into these thematic content units. Gender and ethnic differences were not (usually) topics of intra-group discussion. They were therefore not addressed by coded categories within the texts, but by reconnaissance of group differences over the texts.

TABLE 5.2

Thematic content units

1. Personal meaning of health
2. Concept of time
3. Responsibility for health, power over health
4. Knowledge about health, health and risk behaviour, and consequences
5. Misconceptions about health, health and risk behaviour, and consequences
6. Desired information about health
7. Health behaviours undertaken and justification
8. Risk behaviour undertaken and justification
9. Perceived health and health complaints
10. Attitude, beliefs, feelings concerning general practitioner
11. Self-medication
12. Communication with mother
13. Communication with father
14. Communication with other
15. The ideal self and the experienced self
16. The meaning of the group and peer pressure
17. Resistance and difficulty getting into a topic
18. Rules and authority
19. Dealing with anger, stress, disappointment, and sadness
20. Dealing with examples given by the moderator
21. Meanings or psychological functions of behaviour

The thematic content units were grouped into the five central themes. These form the underlying structure of both the protocol and interview transcripts. The meaning of behaviour, or its subjective psychosocial function, is addressed for every theme.

The central themes are:

- Personal health: meaning, value, personal responsibility and power
- The general practitioner as health counsellor
- Health behaviours: knowledge, behaviour undertaken, and reasons for action
- Risk behaviours: knowledge, behaviour undertaken, and reasons for action
- Autonomy, authority, and health and risk behaviours: breaking the rules.

RESULTS

Personal health: Meaning, value, personal responsibility, and power

When asked directly if the subjects thought much about their health or find it important, the answer was generally no (7 out of 9 groups).

> Health isn't important for me, not really, because my health is good.
> (Turkish/Moroccan girl)

The meaning of health was often expressed in the negative: the meaning of lack of health (8 out of 9 groups). Sickness is "irritating and inconvenient". Health only becomes important when ill health is experienced.

> Health is only important if you get sick, *and*: If you aren't healthy you might get sick.
> (Dutch girl and boy, regular high school)

> Health is important otherwise you can't lead a normal life and you might have a lot of pain. (Dutch boy, college prep.)

> I don't want to go through what my father went through. {Dutch girl, college prep.)

Health also has a social function (all 9 groups).

> If you're not healthy you can't do a lot of things with the other kids, you get left out.
> (Dutch boy, regular high school)

> You can't do anything, can't go to school, get behind on your homework.
> (Dutch girl, regular high school)

The connection between health and many things that the subjects do find important, such as performance in school, sports, or having a good figure was often not made.

> Sport injuries have nothing to do with health. (Dutch boy, regular high school)

The concepts of health over time, or cause and effect, were not well understood. There is a peripheral awareness of now and later, as if in a game. If 'now' is an inconvenient moment to consider health risks, the consideration can be put off until later and the behaviour can take place now. In an almost magical way, this seems to exonerate the risk-taker or exempt her from any unpleasant consequences of her behaviour.

> If I do something that is not good for me, it doesn't really occur to me at the moment. Maybe later I think: 'that was not such a good idea, (Dutch girl and boy, college prep.)

The following anecdote gives another illustration of the multiform concept of time. The topic of childbearing came up in one of the Turkish/Moroccan girls' groups. The discussion centred on career versus children, and the best age for parenthood. After explaining that she wanted to go to school and get a good diploma before she had children, one 15-year-old girl said that she wanted a child when she was 16. She explained this by saying that school was one thing, you are expected to have goals for the future, but on a personal level she just couldn't imagine her life any further away than one year from the time of the interview.

Responsibility for personal health is unanimously shared with the parents.

> If I feel something (in my body), then I have to react to it myself—my mother can't feel what I feel...but my parents carry more responsibility than I do for my health because they say I'm still young, when I'm grown up I'll have to do it myself. But the problem is I don't know when I'll be grown up in their eyes. (Dutch boy, college prep.)

Power over their health, however, is another question. In a discussion on heart disease, when asked if one could avoid it, the answer was no. Medical technology was expected to deal with any (temporary) loss of health:

> There are always medicines and stuff, there are always things that can help. (Dutch boy, regular high school)

Interim conclusions. The adolescents interviewed here do not consider health to be intrinsically important. It is valued only indirectly, for its social function and its contribution to highly valued outcomes such as achievement in school and sports, and to physical attractiveness. However, the relationship between health and these highly valued outcomes is often not perceived by the adolescents. Moreover, adolescents are not yet convinced that they bear responsibility for or power over their own health. This indicates that, while discussion of valued outcomes will certainly get their attention, educational materials which attempt to stimulate health behaviour by emphasising valued outcomes cannot be effective unless an understanding of the principles of cause and effect can be achieved. Understanding health-related principles of cause and effect is often dependent upon an understanding of the passage of time. The adolescents' lack of consistent adherence to the conventional concept of time deprives us of one of our most essential teaching tools. This must be taken into account in the construction of lesson materials for adolescent health education.

The general practitioner as health counsellor

Questions concerning reasons for encounters with the doctor were generally met with resistance and initial silence. Mention of illness or physical trouble of any sort was often accompanied with signs of uneasiness such as coughing and shifting in chairs. Sport injuries, however, seemed easier to discuss in the group situation.

Any contact with the medical world usually goes via the mother (7 out of 9 groups). The general practitioner is, according to these subjects, someone to be avoided (8 out of 9 groups avoid visits to the GP).

> I don't go to the doctor unless they (trainers, parents) say I absolutely have to. (Dutch boy, regular high school)

> I don't like to go, it's unpleasant. (Dutch girl, regular high school)

The overwhelmingly negative attitude towards the GP was related to a lack of confidence in several areas. The doctor was seen as someone who didn't take the time for patients or communicate with them in a way they can understand (6 out of 9 groups).

> You go to the doctor, he shakes your hand, does a little examination, shakes your hand again and you're out of there. You're just a number. (Dutch boy, college prep.)

> Look. If I go to the doctor then you hear that you've got...one or another impossible Latin word, and you don't understand a bit of it. And a little bit of explanation— yeah, like you have a stomach ache because of this or that—well you can FORGET IT! (Dutch boy, regular high school)

The doctor's competence is often doubted and compliance was admittedly low (all 9 groups).

> You go for a headache and he gives you an aspirin and sends you away while it was something else entirely. (Dutch boy, college prep.)

> The doctor doesn't do much anyway. Every doctor says something different (gives a different diagnosis). (Dutch boy, regular high school)

> If I can think of a better way to get over my bronchitis than the spray the doctor gives me that doesn't help anyway, then I'm sure not going to listen to some doctor. (Dutch boy, college prep.)

The adolescents in this sample generally did not feel that they could trust the GP, would never talk to the GP about problems, about body image or sexuality, but only about real 'medical' stuff, and then only sometimes (8 out of 9 groups). They didn't seem to go to the doctor unless they already had an idea of what the problem is, or unless they crossed a particular threshold:

> If I have a vague complaint then I wait to go to the doctor until I think I know what it is, or it is really bad. (Dutch girl, regular high school)

In one of the groups a bit more tolerance was expressed towards the doctor, and more acceptance of the fallibility of medicine:

> Doctors can make mistakes, everyone does. The medicines you get don't always work, but they don't always have to work, so the doctors don't always have to be right. (Dutch boy, regular high school)

Differences between the regular high-school groups and the college prep students in this area were not apparent, nor were differences between girls and boys. There were some cultural differences. The Turkish/Moroccan girls were more open about menstruation in both of the groups. They seemed to have a very clear picture of the changes in medical consumption:

> I hardly ever went to the doctor until I was 14—after that I just seemed to have a lot more complaints, sport injuries at school, bladder infections and stuff. (Turkish/Moroccan girl)

They did not entirely share the general distrust of the doctor exhibited by their Dutch counterparts. The Turkish/Moroccan adolescents in general reported far more visits to the doctor. Complaints include rheumatism, anaemia, and migraine. They went to the doctor more frequently alone and more often at their own initiative, especially if their parents did not speak Dutch. Dutch girls reported more symptoms than the Dutch boys did. This gender difference has been well documented (Pennebaker, 1982; Spruijt-Metz, & Spruijt, 1997). However, the Turkish/Moroccan boys reported more symptoms than the Turkish/Moroccan girls did.

> Girls aren't allowed to complain about their health in our culture. (Turkish/Moroccan girl)

This interaction between gender and ethnicity on symptom report fits with the findings in the questionnaires (Chapter 4).

Interim conclusions. It must be concluded from these results that the general practitioner is not fulfilling a role as first-line health counsellor for these adolescents. This emphasises the need for health education in the schools, and indicates that it should not be assumed that medical information is readily available through the GP. The data also suggests that the problems related to gender and cultural differences in symptom reporting must be reckoned with in the construction of educational materials.

Health behaviours: Knowledge, behaviour undertaken, and reasons for action

When asked to describe healthy behaviours, eating habits were a favourite topic. Every group agreed that one should eat a well-balanced low fat diet at regular mealtimes.

> If I don't eat right or on time mostly I feel sick to my stomach or get a headache or get dizzy and can't concentrate at school ... that's not so good for your grades. (Turkish/Moroccan girl)

The adolescents know a lot about diet, but their knowledge seems to consist of what may be termed 'free-floating facts' about proper and regular diet. Free-floating facts, such as 'fruit and vegetables are good for you' are not embedded in a logically built up network of knowledge, and are often not associated with personal behaviour. For instance, the participants were aware that fatty foods are not healthy, but few foods in this category could be named. It did not seem clear why fatty foods are not healthy, or that this information also pertains to them personally. When asked directly to describe a well balanced diet, many participants could not (7 out of 9 groups) ("What do you mean by 'a healthy diet'?")

> Not going to Macdonald's and stuff. (Dutch girls, college prep.)

Shreds of disorganised information show an accumulation of misunderstandings about nutrition that can best be illustrated by the following exchange, which took place in the girls college prep. group:

> Girl 1: If I eat a lot of sweets, then I eat a whole bunch of apples and then it is okay.
> Girl 2: You shouldn't do that, apples have a lot of sugar in them.
> Girl 3: Yeah, you're better off eating bananas.
> Girl 4: Oh no you're not, bananas are fattening.

This idea that any damage done by a junk food binge could be neutralised by immediately bingeing on a magically equivalent amount of fruit was expressed in four of the groups.

> I eat healthy, like lots of fruit. I also eat a lot of junk food. (Dutch boy, college prep.)

Several healthy behaviours were mentioned, such as exercise, dental hygiene, general hygiene, good posture, getting enough sleep, and talking about your problems. However, the reasons that these behaviours might be healthy are often not understood. For instance, the college prep. boys group unanimously declared that they washed their hands after they go to the bathroom. When asked why washing their hands after visiting the bathroom is healthy, the link from hygiene back to health could not be made:

> For the hygiene, because it's clean and otherwise it's just filthy.

[What does that mean? ... Does it have anything to do with sickness or health?]

No...for me it's purely automatic. I just always do it and I never think about it. (Dutch boy, college prep.)

The knowledge that behaviours are healthy did not necessarily lead to its performance:

Going to bed on time and getting enough sleep is really important. I never do it, though. (Dutch boy, regular high school)

Talking about sex and about problems, or at least expressing your emotions, was mentioned as healthy behaviour in 5 of the 9 groups.

You have to be able to talk about it—that makes everything a lot easier. Otherwise it gets all tied up inside. It is real important, it is a relief. (Dutch boy, regular high school)

However, this knowledge did not lead logically to behaviour.

When I'm sad then I get this lump in my throat and then I don't know what to do, I go up to my room and ... I don't know. I used to cry real hard and then it was over. But now I don't cry anymore and I don't really know what to do... (Dutch boy, college prep.)

The motivations for undertaking healthy behaviours were often unrelated to health (all 9 groups). For instance, the dangers of smoking seemed to be very well understood. It was understood that it is bad for your lungs, addicting, and that those who try to stop may gain weight. However, when asked why they did not smoke, it was not always this knowledge that directed their behaviour, but the personal meaning of the behaviour.

If everybody in the group smokes, then I don't want to ... maybe if nobody did, I would. Whatever, I want to be the opposite. (Dutch boys, regular high school)

And concerning dental hygiene, the following exchange took place in the Dutch boys regular high school group:

Boy 1: Brushing your teeth is real important, I guess. Yeah—but I don't do it very often. Can't be bothered.

Boy 2: I think that as soon as you start going out with a girl, you'll start brushing your teeth!

Interim conclusions. While much information about healthy behaviours seemed to be available to these adolescents, it was not logically structured. Connections between facts were not made, links between behaviour and personal health were frequently unrecognised, and inferences of cause and effect were often misunderstood. Even when these links and connections were made, and causal inferences were understood, behaviour was not necessarily influenced. Undertaking healthy behaviours was more often reported to be related to the meaning with which the behaviours were imbued, and these meanings were often unrelated to health.

Risk behaviours: Knowledge, behaviour undertaken, and reasons for action

The knowledge that the adolescents do have concerning nutrition did not always affect their behaviour.

> Regular diet is real important, but not for me because it doesn't bother me if I don't eat. I mean I don't feel lousy or whatever. (Dutch boy, college prep.)

Body image was urgently important to the girls as well as to the boys (all 9 groups). The boys generally wanted to be more filled out and muscular yet breakfast and lunch were regularly skipped. The girls often find themselves too fat, yet, potato chips, French fries, and sweets were regularly consumed.

> I always have to take sandwiches to school, but I never feel like eating them. I throw them away, and then I'm starving when I get home and eat a whole package of cookies. (Dutch boy, college prep.)

> My mom won't let me go on a diet. She says I should just stop eating sweets and French fries and no more soft drinks and stuff ... but I just can't do it! It has to do with our age ... maybe you're always fat when you're young and then maybe when you get older ... (Dutch girl, college prep.)

Risky eating behaviour often had a meaning or function that was very well articulated, as shown by this exchange between the interviewer and a Dutch boy from the regular high-school group:

> If I eat too little for a long time, my stomach shrinks, and then if I eat a lot then it feels ... then I know it is real bad if you don't eat regularly.

> [Why do you do it, then?]

> ...Well...I'm just not going to adjust to their [parents] mealtimes.

Food consumption was regularly influenced by moods (8 of 9 groups). Several meanings (or functions) of behaviour were mentioned in this context, such as eating sweets or junk food as a way to 'spoil' yourself, food as comfort, bingeing as a way to be aggressive towards yourself, and eating (or starving) as a way to deal with anger, frustration, or 'feeling down':

> It just depends on my mood—Sometimes I'm in a certain mood and then I think— "what do I care"—and I just throw my lunch away. Sometimes I think about it—that I would like to be more muscular and stuff, then I'm in the sort of a mood that I look in the mirror a lot and stuff—and then I eat my lunch. (Dutch boy, college prep.)

> If I'm sad then I can't eat, or if I'm nervous. But if I'm angry—boy, then I eat bags full of liquorice! (Dutch boy, college prep.)

> I'm always sorry afterwards—if I'm like angry or feel sorry for myself, I buy a giant bag of sweets and eat it all up ... and then a half an hour later I think "oh shit", or if I see a cute guy at school then I think why did I do that because now I'm too fat. Then I hate myself, then I'm ashamed. (Dutch girl, regular high school)

Risky behaviours were often an expression of anger or impatience, which appeared to have a mitigating effect on their risky character:

> My father is really concerned about my health—so if I'm really mad at my father and stuff and it's winter and real cold then I go outside without a coat on. (Dutch boy, college prep.)

> If I'm pissed off then I turn on my Walkman real loud—that makes my father real angry. I know it's bad for my ears, so it is okay. (Dutch boys, college prep.)

> I usually bike through red traffic lights—I just don't feel like waiting. (Dutch girl, college prep.)

Risky behaviour seems to be an imperative:

> You've just got to, man. (Turkish/Moroccan boy)

Although there were no apparent gender differences in the amount of reported risk behaviour, the type of behaviour seemed to differ. Girls were more likely to turn to food, especially sweets, when feeling sad or frustrated (all 6 groups in which girls participated), whereas boys reported more unsafe sports, listening to loud music, going to sleep late, or disobeying of rules when angry or frustrated.

There were several cultural differences. It was comparatively more difficult to get the Turkish/Moroccan boys to honestly discuss risky behaviours. The influence of Islam in the lives of the Turkish/Moroccan girls generated a category of behaviour that they themselves considered risky for their general health. This had to do with any sport (such as bicycling) or the use of tampons, which they feared might cause rupture of the hymen.

Interim conclusions. The adolescents' information on risk behaviours did not seem to be organised into a rational network of knowledge upon which reasonable action can be based, nor did it seem to directly discourage risky behaviour. Even when connections were understood between abstaining from risky behaviour and a valued outcome (for instance decreasing sweets intake and weight loss), behaviour was not necessarily influenced. Once again, the meanings with which behaviours were imbued were reported to influence behaviour most directly. These meanings eclipsed both knowledge and desires for valued outcomes. The particular meaning with which a behaviour is imbued may be influenced by gender and by cultural background.

Autonomy, authority, and health and risk behaviours: Breaking the rules

Autonomy and individuation are major focuses in adolescence (Cobb, 1992; Erikson, 1963). These themes were also dominant in the interviews. Breaking the rules, challenging authority, and the conflict between making one's own rules and following those laid down by others were often indicated as meanings and determinants of behaviour:

> If my mother says I'm not allowed [to eat candy, or stay out too late]—then sometimes I just do it to show that I'm right. (Turkish/Moroccan girl)

The role of risk-taking in testing your own limits was mentioned in most groups (8 out of 9 groups):

> My health is important, sure, but sometimes I do dangerous things, break the rules because it scares me ... deep in my heart I'm afraid that something will go wrong, that I'll get hurt or get caught ... but that's really exciting ... and you can think back on it later, and say to yourself ... 'I did that!' (Dutch girl, regular high school)

Breaking rules and taking risks have limits as well as functions that are clearly understood and eloquently stated:

> You break the rules so that afterwards you can make your own choices. (Dutch girl, college prep.)

> It gives me a kick, makes me feel free ... to lie to my parents and stay out real late ... and fool them. But you can't do it too often. Otherwise you don't ... respect your parents anymore ... or they won't trust you ... and then you end out just fooling yourself. (Dutch girl, regular high school)

After treating us to a technical explanation of how he regulated the lighting in his room and used his hockey stick to turn his TV on and off so that he could stay up late and watch TV after his parents had forbidden it, one boy offered the following explanation for his behaviour:

> It feels good to break the rules, it's exciting, even if I know I'll feel lousy in the morning. And it is part of life, you have to show that you're free, that you can do what you want, that you are in control. (Dutch boy, college prep.)

One boy told of his regular dangerous behaviour on his bike on the way to school:

> I need the adventure, the challenge.

> [But I don't get it, some rules you all seem to break, others you don't ...]

> Breaking some rules makes you a better person, breaking others doesn't, that's all. Riding like a madman on my bike, for instance, that gives me self-confidence. And then you feel better about yourself and that's real important. (Dutch boy, regular high school)

Interim conclusions. A complex of meanings that guide behaviour in adolescence emerged around issues concerning autonomy, authority, and testing personal limits within society. While the behaviours that become associated with these meanings were often unhealthy or dangerous, the meanings in and of themselves had long been accepted as belonging to the process of human development. Many of the adolescents in the focus groups expressed inner limits concerning risk behaviours, a point at which risk behaviours become disassociated from salient meanings. Breaking some rules was considered beneficial, breaking others was considered foolish, and breaking the 'breakable' ones too often overshot the goal, disassociating the behaviour from the original meaning.

DISCUSSION

The primary role that the affective meaning of a behaviour may assume as a determinant of that behaviour was central to the findings in these interviews. According to the data, personal meanings often guide behaviour and overrule health-related knowledge and values. Behaviours may mean a way of enhancing the self-image, of expressing rebellion, of dealing with anger, frustration, nervousness, impatience, or sadness. Health and risk behaviours become ways of comforting, rewarding, and punishing oneself. Both health and risk behaviours often emanate from implicit or explicit rules, and undertaking them often involves obedience/disobedience or compliance/non-compliance with parents or other authority figures. Through this, behaviour takes on meanings of individuation, exercising personal will, assuming or rejecting personal responsibility, testing personal boundaries, and challenging authority. As adolescents teeter on the boundary between dependence and independence, the meanings that behaviours assume often reflect this vacillation. Some behaviours represent the demand for the freedom to assume responsibility for their own bodies, while other behaviours— or even the same behaviours in different contexts, represent refusal to accept that responsibility.

Behaviours are imbued with meanings that are often totally unrelated to the 'cause and effect' type of knowledge-based meanings subscribed to by parents, teachers, and doctors. This is, in a way, not surprising. The cause and effect relationships between health and health behaviour are spread out in time, oblique and difficult to understand even for many adults (Pennebaker, 1990). While much information is available to these adolescents, it has not yet been incorporated into a solid body of abstract ideas that allow generalisation to similar situations and replace magical thinking. Even when concrete and correct knowledge is available, it is often no match for the more affective meanings with which behaviour is empowered by the adolescent. While different levels of cognitive development are represented in the groups interviewed here, they did not seem to differ in the lack of a consistent, logically built up, accessible, and functional network of knowledge on health and risk behaviours.

The behavioural and social outcomes of health have been found to be salient in adolescents' health concept (Shiloh, & Waiser, 1991). In this sample, although health does not appear to be intrinsically valued, several social and behavioural outcomes of health are, such as school attendance and sport achievements. The lack of connections made between healthy behaviour and valued outcomes seems related to the adolescents' singular experience of time, which does not yet flow in a steady, chronological fashion and retains some magical properties. The impermanence of the passage of time in this conceptualisation implies that any harm done to personal health through risk-taking or neglect is reversible or inconceivably distant in time. In the development of health education materials for healthy adolescents, understanding of their conceptualisations of health and time should be utilised to formulate effective communications.

One major advantage of the focus group methodology for this research was the ideas generated in group discussions. The general level of excitement over the topic eventually drew every member of each group into the discussion. The extreme delicacy of health-related issues when talking on a personal level, however, had not been foreseen. Resistance had to be overcome in every group and covert taboos concerning all things physical had to be confronted repeatedly. Health-related issues touch upon many sensitive areas. These must be dealt with in a fashion that does not provoke resistance. This will need to be taken into account in the construction of lesson materials.

The qualitative nature of this study did not allow for testing the hypothesis that meanings of behaviour are determinants of health and risk behaviour in adolescence. The relationship between behaviours and their meanings was conceived of as personal in nature, not necessarily logical or rational in any collective sense. Whether group interview techniques could be used to generate valid and reliable information concerning personal meanings of behaviour now needed to be examined. To do this, the next step would be to use the focus group transcripts for the construction of survey materials. Quantitative hypothesis testing now needed to be conducted. The interview data showed that further research into the development of associations between meanings and health and risk behaviours in adolescence was warranted.

Meanings are imbedded in culture. In this study, some behaviours took on entirely different meanings for the Turkish/Moroccan groups than for the Dutch group. Gender differences were also apparent, especially in meanings of behaviour relating to nutrition. These differences in meanings attributed to behaviour will need to be taken into account in the design of the next phase of the research and further explored.

In this study, the meaning of behaviour emerged as a primary determinant for both health and risk behaviours in adolescence. These deeply rooted affective meanings subsume health-related knowledge and values. As I saw it, research into the development and nature of associations between meanings and behaviours could offer the potential to help adolescents make and break these associations through education, allowing salient meanings to be linked with functional behaviours. While methods of incorporation of these meanings into lesson materials still needed to be explored, making connections between meanings and knowledge, and bringing these meanings to the foreground could serve an interesting function:

> During my adolescence, asthma attacks became a routine feature of the windy part of winter. Clearly, I reasoned, pollen and dust ... were to blame. In college, I never had any wheezing bouts except when I went home for the Christmas holidays ... All of a sudden, the profound realisation hit me that there was more to my asthma than pollen. Conflicts with my parents were undoubtedly the link to my upper respiratory system. Interestingly, once I saw the parent–asthma connection, I never again wheezed. It was too embarrassing. (Pennebaker, 1990)

It seemed that the understanding of the meanings with which behaviours are invested could offer a valuable tool for the creation of effective health education materials.

PART THREE

Quantitative studies: Formulating theory and understanding adolescent health

CHAPTER SIX

Worries and health in adolescence[1]

Co-author: Rob J. Spruijt

INTRODUCTION

The qualitative phase of the research had been completed, and it was time to adopt a more quantitative approach in order to test hypotheses that had been developed. In this quantitative phase, a large-scale survey was administered in numerous school districts throughout The Netherlands. The questionnaire was designed by amalgamating the knowledge gathered in the first, theoretical phase of the research and the data gathered in the second, qualitative phase of the research. The analysis of the abundance of data provided by this survey was partitioned into three segments. These are presented in the next three chapters (6, 7, and 8).

Five specific goals had been set in Chapter 4: (1) to appraise current knowledge about health in the Dutch adolescent population, (2) to inventory perceived health and take stock of the health complaints of the group, (3) to assess health and risk behaviours adolescents undertake, (4) to explore the feasibility of reaching different cultural groups with the same material, and (5) to uncover possible determinants of health and risk behaviour. These, taken together with the overall goal of developing relevant and effective lesson materials, informed the development of the questionnaire and the subsequent analysis of the data. This chapter looks at the data pertaining to the second goal and to the relevance criterion. Here we will look at how adolescents perceive their own health and the nature of their most frequent health complaints. We also will explore the nature of the target groups' most salient

[1]Parts of this chapter appeared previously as: Spruijt-Metz, D., & Spruijt, R. (1997). Worries and health in adolescence: A latent variable approach. *Journal of Youth and Adolescence, 26*(4), 485–501. Reprinted by permission of Plenum Press.

121

concerns or 'worries', and investigate the relationship between perceived health and these worries.

The 'worry' construct had proven to be an interesting and useful one in the focus groups, sparking many discussions. Data from the focus group interviews suggested that health was related to worries obliquely, if not directly. It seemed that an understanding of the content and correlates of adolescents' worries might provide pivotal information on their life styles, problems, and interests (Van Asselt, & Lanphen, 1990; Cluitmans, Gouwenberg, & Miltenburg, 1989; Hamilton, Whitney, & Sizer, 1991; McGuire, Mitic, & Neumann, 1987; Orton, 1982; Wadden, Brown, Foster, & Linowitz, 1991). If salient worries could capture the target groups' imagination and interest, and these worries were related to health, then developing an in-depth understanding of adolescent worries might contribute to both the relevance and effectiveness of health education materials. The study of worries could uncover motivating factors for target behaviours and help to interconnect subject matter and teaching approaches with the interests and needs of the target group. The act of worrying might also have a direct effect on health.

'Worries' have been defined as "intrusive, affectively-laden thoughts and images" (Borkovec, Robinson, Pruzinsky, & DePree, 1983) and refer to inner processes which may or may not be related to real events in the environment (Kaufman et al., 1993; Orton, 1982). Worries are related to daily hassles, most clearly to the 'inner concerns' factor reflected in daily hassles measurement as described by Lazarus et al. (1985). Hassles have been defined as "mundane irritants and sources of stress that people commonly encounter in everyday life" (Kohn, & Milrose, 1993). Several studies have linked daily hassles to reduced health in adolescent populations (Kanner, Feldman, Weinberger, & Ford, 1987; Wu, & Lam, 1993). The conceptual association between daily hassles and worries suggests that worries may also be stressors linked to negative health outcomes. However, when predicting subjective well-being from exposure to stressors such as daily hassles or worries, it can be contended that the measure directly reflects those aspects of negative well-being it is intended to predict. Dohrenwend and Shrout (1985) argue that the measurement of daily hassles is confounded with symptoms of psychological distress such as negative affectivity. The problem of confusion between independent and dependent variables can be approached by attempting to generate a decontaminated measure, as has been done for life events (Dohrenwend, & Shrout, 1985; Schroeder, & Costa, 1984) and daily hassles (Kohn, & Milrose, 1993). A theoretically attractive alternative is to simultaneously examine the separate contributions of negative affectivity and worries to variation in physiological status, as Whitehead (1994) has suggested for life event and daily hassles measurement. Extrapolation of this alternative invites the postulation that both negative affectivity and perceived exposure to stressors are indicators of one underlying construct, together with other related indicators. Weiss, Weiss, Politano, and Carey (1991) report a strong relationship between fatigue and affective disturbances in adolescents. Fatigue also affects adolescents' perception of their physiological well-being (Tynjala, Kannas, & Valimaa, 1993). Both feelings of loneliness and the perceived quality of parental relationships show strong relationships to overall perceived psychosocial well-being (Spruijt-Metz, 1996). Parental relationships, depending upon their positive or negative nature, can play a prominent role in either buffering or exacerbating perceived stress and hassles (Hurrelmann, Uwe, & Weidman, 1992). A constellation of indicators emerges including worries, affect, fatigue, and relational variables denoting one underlying construct that might be termed 'psychosocial well-being', which appears to be related to health perceptions.

Structural Equation Modelling (SEM) provides a fine tool for examining relationships between complex constructs without having to look at each 'path' separately. With SEM, you can test an entire model at once. SEM not only tests the hypotheses concerning relationships between constructs. It also tests the quantification of the underlying constructs (known in SEM as latent variables). In SEM, latent variables are defined as the simultaneous effect of several observed variables. Using this methodology, the relationship between psychosocial well-being and health or physiological status can be examined. Structural modelling of the relationship between psychosocial well-being and physiological status also permits closer examination of the repeated findings that girls report more hassles (Kanner et al., 1987), more stressful life-events (Hotaling, Atwell, & Linsky, 1978; Newcomb, Huba, & Bentler, 1981), more worries (Kaufman et al., 1993; Klingman, 1998; McGuire et al., 1987; Orton, 1982; Vervaet, van Heeringen, & Jannes, 1998), more symptoms (Pennebaker, 1982; Settertobulte, & Kolip, 1997; Spruijt, & Spruijt-Metz, 1994; Spruijt-Metz et al., 1994), more negative affectivity (Watson, & Pennebaker, 1989), and poorer health (Netherlands Central Bureau of Statistics, 1992) than boys.

In this chapter, the findings from the data on salient worries and health complaints in adolescence are described and incorporated into a structural model of the relationship between psychosocial well-being and physiological status. This relationship is examined, and the meaning of gender differences in this context is explored.

Box 6.1: A brief word on Structural Equation Modelling (SEM)

Structural Equation Modelling (also known as Structural Modelling or Linear Structural Equation Modelling) is a data analysis technique that subsumes both latent variable analysis, factor analysis and path analysis. SEM provides a test of the viability of any model as a whole, all at once, simultaneously. This means that if you used, let's say, the theory of Reasoned Action (see Chapter 3) in your research and have accrued the appropriate data, you can test the degree to which the TRA really fits your data (or is applicable to your sample) in one fell swoop using SEM! This technique offers a number of advantages over its predecessors, which required multiple testing and the separate interpretation of each relationship in a model.

Box 6.1 continued

Box 6.1: A brief word on Structural Equation Modelling (SEM) (continued)

The three major statistical packages that test structural equation models are LISREL (Jöreskog, 1973; Jöreskog, & Sörbom, 1986), EQS (Bentler, 1986; Bentler, & Weeks, 1980), and AMOS (Arbuckle, 1997). All three packages use slightly different terminology for their models, which can be confusing and irritating, but the principal is basically the same. Lists of other software packages that run structural models along with much other information on SEM can be found on the World Wide Web (for instance: West, 1999). There is also a journal devoted entirely to SEM, *Structural Equation Modelling*, published by Lawrence Erlbaum Associates. We used LISREL for the analyses in this chapter.

Bollen (1989) identifies three components in SEM: (1) path analysis, (2) a conceptual synthesis of latent variable and measurement models, and (3) general estimation procedures. What does this mean?

Path analysis: SEM tells you the strength of the relationship between each of the latent and observed variables included in your model. In other words, SEM analyses all the paths between variables at once. It allows you to distinguish direct, indirect and total effects of one variable upon another for all variables in a given model. Let's say we want to know how well the theory of Reasoned Action predicts smoking. SEM can calculate the effect of attitudes towards smoking upon actual smoking behaviour, the indirect effect of attitudes on smoking (via other variables such as intention), and the total effect (direct plus indirect) of attitudes upon smoking. SEM does this all at once, without having to test each path separately, taking all effects (and error) into account, and giving a complete picture of all the paths.

Observed and latent variables: SEM makes a distinction between observed variables and latent variables. Observed variables are what you actually measure, your operationalisations. Latent variables are the constructs these operationalisations are meant to represent. SEM examines both a measurement model and a structural model. The indices for the measurement model tell you the extent to which your observed variables or operationalisations (questions, items, questionnaires, observations, etc.) form indicators for your latent variable (attitude, intention, behaviour, and so forth). Examination of the measurement model using SEM essentially yields factor loadings, rather like factor analysis. It tells you if the various operationalisations chosen to represent 'attitude' in your bit of research on smoking can really be said to represent the latent variable. SEM examines not only the viability of your measurements; it also examines the viability of the underlying theory. To do this, SEM examines the structural model, which is the relationship between latent variables. This takes us one step further than path analysis and factor analysis combined.

General estimation procedures: SEM can deliver several different estimations of goodness of fit of the structural model to your data. To continue with the example concerning the TRA and smoking, these estimations allow us to determine the extent to which attitude (a latent, unobserved variable that is represented by our operationalisations) really affects behaviour (another latent, unobserved variable represented by our operationalisations). In other words, SEM will tell you if the TRA, in its entirety, as represented by your operationalisations, really says something informative about the data that you have accrued (i.e. if it 'fits' your data).

METHODS

Sample

The results from the qualitative round indicated that lesson materials for Turkish, Moroccan, and other immigrant youth required separate and intensive study and in-depth understanding of their cultures and the affects of acculturation (Berry, Poortinga, & Pandey, 1997). To include them marginally would not do them justice, nor would it contribute to our understanding of their needs. Therefore, it was decided to complete this study with predominantly Dutch subjects and plan future studies with the immigrant and minority populations. This decision rendered the fourth goal (to explore the feasibility of reaching different cultural groups with the same material) a moot point. The preliminary data indicated that different cultural groups could not be reached effectively using the same educational materials.

Based upon the clear cognitive differences between the vocational and college preparatory high school students and the advice of educational material publishers, the choice was made to proceed exclusively with college preparatory high-school students. A total of 416 high-school students (211 girls and 205 boys), primarily with a Dutch background, took part in this study (described in this and the following two chapters). The ages of the subjects varied from 11 to 18, with a mean age of 14. The sample was drawn from six secondary schools in five different regions in The Netherlands. The students were requested to fill in a questionnaire during class. Completion of the questionnaire took about 45 minutes, or one class period.

The questionnaire consisted of three sections (with some overlap). One section was on worries and other psychosocial variables, one on perceived health, and one on health-related behaviours and their determinants. Results from each of the three sections of the questionnaire are reported on here in separate chapters. Some of the measurements (for instance, the health complaint index) were used in more than one analysis. Therefore, Chapters 6, 7, and 8 share a common sample, and have some variables in common.

Independent variables: Psychosocial well-being

The exogenous latent variable 'psychosocial well-being' was indicated by five observed variables: the worry list, an affect scale, a measure of ease of communication with parents, a tiredness measure and a loneliness measure.

The worry list represents the 13 most salient worries of Dutch adolescents. While several inventories of adolescent concerns have been constructed (for instance: Alexander, 1989; Compas, 1993; Dohrenwend, & Shrout, 1985; Hamilton, Van Mouwerik, Oetting, Beauvais, & Keilin, 1988; Kohn, & Milrose, 1993; Lazarus, 1984; McGuire et al., 1987; Newcomb et al., 1981; Orton, 1982; Wu, & Lam, 1993), the salience of adolescent worries and concerns are dependent upon culture and influenced by *Zeitgeist* (Kaufman et al., 1993; Nurmi, Poole, & Kalakoski, 1994).

Therefore, a new list was constructed for this study. This was done by combining data from the focus group interviews and data from the pilot questionnaire (consisting of 12 items and an open question), in which Dutch adolescents were asked to describe their most salient worries in their own words (Spruijt-Metz, & Spruijt, 1997; Chapters 4 and 5 of this book). Thirteen worries were incorporated into the worry list used in this study. The worry list shows good internal consistency (Cronbach's alpha = .79 for the entire sample, .80 for the girls, .73 for the boys), and examination of the scree plot of eigenvalues from a maximum likelihood factor analysis with varimax rotation suggests that a one-factor solution best fits the data. The worry list serves to quantify worrying by giving an indication of how much or how often adolescents worry and to rank the worries in order of importance. Each item is scored on a Likert scale ranging from 1 (I never worry about this) to 5 (I often worry about this).

The affect scale (Cronbach's alpha = .72 for the entire sample, .69 for the girls, .74 for the boys) is a three-item scale, representing an abbreviation of the measurement for affectivity used by Watson and Pennebaker (1989). Frequency of bad moods, feeling 'rotten', and feeling nervous are scored on a five-point scale (1= never to 5 = often). A high score on the affectivity scale indicates high negative affect.

Ease of communication with parents was assessed by asking if the subjects found it easy to talk about troublesome or important things with parents or caretakers. A score of 0 indicates that the subject cannot communicate with either parent, a score of 1 indicates that the subject can communicate with one parent, and a score of 2 indicates ease of communication with both parents. Frequency of feeling tired or lethargic in the morning was measured on a four-point scale (1 = never to 4 = often), as was frequency of feeling lonely.

Dependent variables: Physiological status

The endogenous latent variable 'physiological status' was indicated by four observed variables: a global self-rated health item, a symptom checklist, the frequency of doctors' visits in the last half year, and the frequency of aspirin use.

The global health status item is a rating of personal health on a five point scale (1 = very good to 5 = very poor). The global health measure is often used as a health indicator and has been shown to be a valid measure (Krause, & Jay, 1994).

The PILL (Pennebaker Inventory of Limbic Languidness; Pennebaker, 1982) is a symptom checklist, which measures the overall tendency to report symptoms. The Dutch translation has been used by Spruijt and Spruijt-Metz (1994) and van Vliet (1992). Respondents rated the frequency with which they are bothered by each of 52 symptoms on a five-point scale (1 = never, 5 = frequently). The PILL (Cronbach's alpha = .92 for the entire sample, .90 for the girls, .91 for the boys) was used here to rank symptoms according to prevalence among adolescents, to assess the tendency to report symptoms, and as an indicator of health status.

While subjective complaint scales contain a valid, health-related component, use in conjunction with other indicators of health status, such as behavioural measures, has been advised (Watson, & Pennebaker, 1989). The behaviours chosen as general health indicators are frequency of doctors' visits and frequency of aspirin use. Frequency of doctors' visits within the last half-year was assessed by self-report. Aspirin consumption was assessed on a five point scale (1 = never to 5 = four or more times a week) (also self-reported).

Data analysis

The five predictor and four criterion variables were examined for gender differences with t-tests and χ^2 tests for independence. Additionally, salient worries and physical symptoms were ranked according to mean scores. Spearman's rank correlation coefficient was used to uncover possible gender differences in the rankings of worries and symptoms.

The model of the relationship between psychosocial well-being and physiological status, shown in Fig. 6.1, was tested using structural equation modelling (LISREL 8).

The measurement part of the model depicted here asserts that worry, affect, parental communication, tiredness and loneliness are indicators of one underlying latent variable: psychosocial well being. It also asserts that self-rated health, the PILL, frequency of doctors' visits, and aspirin consumption are indicators of another underlying latent variable: physiological status. The structural part of the model asserts that psychosocial well being is a determinant of physiological status. Other possible determinants not studied here are summarised in the model as zeta (ζ), or error.

Multi-sample model testing and nested modelling techniques were combined to examine the tenability of the proposed model for both girls and boys (Bollen, 1989). Gender differences in parameter estimates were studied by examining three increasingly restrictive nested versions of the models, versions A, B, and C. In

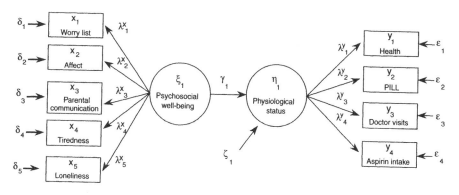

FIG. 6.1   Model of the relationship between psychosocial well-being and physiological status.

version A of the model, the hypothesis concerning the general *form* of the overall model is tested. This hypothesis states that the general model fits for both girls and boys without putting any restraints on measurement or structural parameters (represented by arrows marked with lambda (λ) and gamma (γ) respectively in Fig. 6.1). Thus, this version does not require that the values of the parameters be similar for boys and girls. If and only if this hypothesis cannot be rejected, can the second hypothesis be tested. The second hypothesis states that, given the first hypothesis, the measurement model is the same for both girls and boys. The measurement model refers to the factor structure of the latent variables (the parameters representing the measurement model are marked with a λ). Technically speaking, in version B the parameters pertaining to the measurement model are constrained to be invariant over both groups while the structural parameter, which connects the latent variables and is marked with a γ, is allowed to vary. Invariance of measurement models between boys and girls indicates that the relation between the observed variables and the underlying latent variables can be assumed to be the same in both groups. This implies that the latent variables can be interpreted in the same way for both groups. Spruijt (1994) has shown that this is a prerequisite for meaningful interpretations of relationships between the latent variables (the structural model, marked with γ). Therefore, only if the second hypothesis cannot be rejected, can Version C be tested. This hypothesis states that, given hypotheses 1 and 2, the structural model (in this case, the parameter marked by the γ), is the same for boys and girls. Here, all parameters are invariant, including the relationship between the two latent variables. This is the most restrictive model. As we proceed through the three increasingly restrictive models, we place more stringent requirements on our data at each step. Each step must be completed successfully, otherwise testing the next assumption is no longer meaningful. In version A, we test the overall form of the model for its credibility as a representation of the data. In version B, by comparing the reduction of observed variables to latent variables, the hypothesis that the latent variables have the same interpretation in both groups is tested. In version C, the theoretically most interesting hypothesis, whether these latent variables are related in the same way for both groups, is tested.

Because the analysis involves mixed continuous and ordinal measurements, the asymptotically distribution free weighted least squares (WLS) estimation procedure was needed (Bollen, 1989). As is recommended for this situation involving mixed measurement levels, a matrix of polychoric, polyserial, and Pearson correlations among the indicators was generated using PRELIS, as well as the asymptotic variance-covariance matrix of correlations needed for the WLS estimation procedure (Jöreskog, 1990).

RESULTS

The data were examined for multivariate outliers on the predictor and criteria variables by requesting Mahalanobis D^2 (Tabachnick, & Fidell, 1996). Mahalanobis distance quantifies the (multivariate) distance of any subject from the combined means of the sample on the variables included in the analysis. Eight outlying cases were identified at an alpha = .01 cut-off level and were deleted from the analysis (Stevens, 1992). A significant Mahalanobis D^2 indicates that the subject's response pattern is atypical, and may not be representative of the sample. The outliers were not systematically identified with either gender or with a particular age group, and were characterised by maximum scores on loneliness, the worry list or the PILL. Five girls and nine boys were omitted due to missing data. The analyses were carried out using data from the remaining 394 cases.

Examination of the observed variables revealed numerous gender differences, as shown in Table 6.1. The power of these tests is high because of the relatively large sample size and therefore measures of effect size (d for t-tests and w for χ^2 statistic) are included to improve interpretability of the results (Cohen, 1988). Two significant results show small effects (perceived health and number of doctor visits). The remaining significant differences show medium or large effect sizes, suggesting that the significances reflect substantial differences. Girls and boys differed on six of the nine variables, with the girls reporting more worries, more negative affectivity, more symptoms, more doctors' visits and more aspirin use. The boys report better health.

Figure 6.2 shows the hierarchy of worries for girls and boys. Although girls generally worry more than boys do, their priorities are similar. 'Love' is at the top of both lists, 'health' is at the bottom of both lists (Spearman's r_s = .71, p = .01).

In Fig. 6.3, the top 10 symptoms of the 52-symptom PILL are ranked in descending order for both girls and boys. The mean PILL score is higher for girls than for boys, however the symptom rankings for the 52 items are comparable (Spearman's r_s = .89, p = .00). Here, as in the statistics for the worry list, is evidence

TABLE 6.1

Descriptive statistics, t-tests, and χ2 statistics concerning gender differences on the observed variables

Variable	Girls (n=201)		Boys (n=193)			
	Mean	(SD)	Mean	(SD)	t-value	d
x_1 Worry list	2.11	(.58)	1.81	(.49)	5.49**[a]	.55
x_2 Affect scale	2.53	(.79)	2.11	(.80)	5.28**	.53
x_4 Tiredness	2.90	(.77)	2.75	(.98)	1.69[a]	.17
x_5 Loneliness	1.64	(.67)	1.69	(1.01)	−.59[a]	.05
y_1 Health	4.13	(.79)	4.39	(.71)	−3.38**	.35
y_2 PILL	1.83	(.38)	1.56	(.34)	7.44**	.75
y_3 Doctor visits	1.95	(2.37)	1.29	(1.82)	3.12**[a]	.31
y_4 Aspirin intake	2.21	(.84)	1.73	(.71)	6.10**[a]	.62
x_3 Parental communication	χ^2 = 7.95		df = 2		p = .02	w = .38

**p <.01

[a]Behrens-Fisher solution for separate variance estimates employed because variances differed at p<.05.

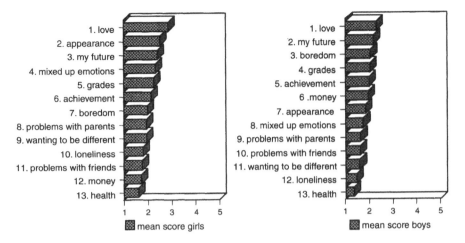

FIG. 6.2   Worries ranked in order of priority for girls and boys.

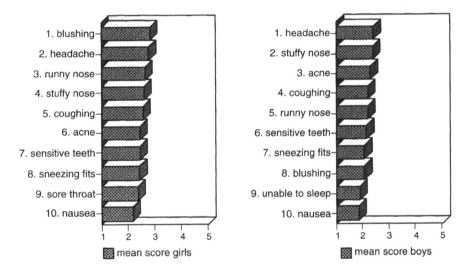

FIG. 6.3   Girls' and boys' 'top ten' highest ranking symptoms.

that the gender differences often observed in worries, hassles, symptom report and the like may not be qualitative differences, but quantitative differences of degree.

Corrections for deviations from multivariate normality were carried out in PRELIS. The correlation matrix generated by PRELIS is shown in Table 6.2.

Various measures of fit can be used to evaluate the fit between structural model equations and the data (Tanaka, 1993). Brief descriptions of the measures cited in

TABLE 6.2

Correlations between the observed variables

	Worry	Affect	Parents	Tired	Lonely	Health	PILL	Doctor	Aspirin
x_1 Worry	—	.483	−.328	.240	.175	−.297	.487	.082	.103
x_2 Affect	.650	—	−.148	.203	.116	−.219	.513	.128	.178
x_3 Parents	−.172	−.177	—	−.203	−.094	.155	−.170	−.049	−.071
x_4 Tired	.324	.311	−.100	—	.047	−.189	.233	.025	.112
x_5 Lonely	.496	.347	.019	.062	—	−.117	.188	.041	.026
y_1 Health	−.327	−.338	.077	−.141	−.211	—	−.358	−.185	−.191
y_2 PILL	.567	.608	−.094	.348	.281	−.373	—	.155	.194
y_3 Doctor	.139	.158	.043	.145	.004	−.263	.264	—	.068
y_4 Aspirin	.260	.292	−.037	.112	.095	−.283	.318	.171	—

Correlation for girls ($n = 201$) are below the diagonal of the matrix
Correlation for boys ($n = 193$) are above the diagonal of the matrix

Table 6.3 are given in Box 6.2, along with summaries of their anticipated performance for nested models.

It must be said that the indices discussed in Box 6.2 do not test one model against another. Choosing the best fitting model using goodness of fit indices is a question

---

Box 6.2: Some estimation procedures offered by LISREL

♦ The likelihood-ratio chi-square measure of fit should be non-significant, demonstrating that there is no significant discrepancy between the observed and the predicted covariance matrices.

♦ The RMSEA (Root Means Square Error of Approximation) takes the error of approximation in the population and the precision of the fit measure itself into account. It is a measure of discrepancy per degree of freedom. A RMSEA of < .05 indicates a close fit.

♦ The EVCI (Expected Cross-Validation Index), the AIC (Akaike Information Criterion), and the CAIC (Corrected Akaike Information Criterion) compare models on the basis of criteria that take parsimony (the number of parameters) into account as well as fit. For these three indices, the model with the smallest value is considered to have the best fit.

♦ The GFI (Goodness of Fit Index) does not depend on sample size and measures how much better the model fits as compared to no model at all. This index should be .90 or higher for an adequate model.

♦ The NFI (Normed Fit Index), the NNFI (Non-Normed Fit Index), the CFI (Comparative Fit Index) and the IFI (Incremental Fit Index) measure how much better the model fits compared to a baseline model, usually the independence model. The value of these indices often approaches 1 for a well-fitting model.

♦ The PGFI (Parsimony Goodness of Fit Index) and the PNFI (Parsimony Normed Fit Index) compare model fit to baseline models, but also take parsimony into account. The value of these indices goes up as the number of parameters goes down.

TABLE 6.3

Summary of the goodness-of-fit indices for the models

Index	Model A Hform (all parameters free)	Model B Hmeasurement ($\lambda x, \lambda y, \theta\delta, \theta\varepsilon$ constrained)	Model C Hstructure (all parameters constrained)	Model C Hstructure-ϕ (all parameters constrained except Phi (ϕ), variance of psychosocial well-being)
$\chi 2$ (df) p	61.41 (52) .17	79.88 (68) .15	88.62 (71) .08	81.37 (70) .17
RMSEA	.021	.021	.025	.020
EVCI	.35	.32	.32	.31
AIC	137.41	123.88	126.62	121.37
CAIC	326.51	233.36	221.17	220.89
GFI	.97	.96	.96	.96
NFI	.91	.89	.87	.88
NNFI	.98	.98	.97	.98
CFI	.99	.98	.97	.98
IFI	.99	.98	.97	.98
PGFI	1.12	1.45	1.51	1.49
PNFI	.66	.84	.86	.86
		Model B vs. Model A	Model C vs. Model B	Model ϕ free vs. Model B
D^2 (df)		18.47 (16)	8.74 (3)	1.49 (3)
Significance		NS	Sig. at $P = .05$	NS

of interpreting patterns of values and the changes in those patterns between different models. When nested model methodology is applied, there are measures available to test one model against another. The likelihood ratio test statistic (D^2) is one such measure (Jöreskog, & Sörbom, 1993). D^2 is the absolute difference in χ^2 values of two nested models and is itself χ^2 distributed. Degrees of freedom for D^2 are equal to the absolute difference in degrees of freedom of the χ^2 values for the two models being tested. If D^2 is significant, the model with fewer parameters does not offer an improvement over the less parsimonious model, regardless of the fit.

In Table 6.3, the goodness of fit indices and D^2 are summarised for Model A, Model B, and Model C. While all models fit, D^2 is significant between Model B and Model C. Also, the ECVI remains equal and the AIC increases between models B and C, whereas a decrease in these indices are indicators of improved fit. Examination of the modification indices provided by LISREL 8 suggested stress in the estimate of the variance of psychosocial well being (ϕ). A fourth model was generated, Model C′, in which only phi (ϕ) is unconstrained and all other parameters are invariant over the two groups. Statistics for this model are also given in Table 6.3.

The fourth model, Model C′, proves to be the best model. D^2 is not significant between Model B and Model C′, in which phi (ϕ) is free. The EVCI and the AIC both decrease between the two models, and most of the other fit indices indicate a better fit for the fourth model. In the best fitting model, the general form of the model and the measurement model are the same for girls and boys, and the structural model holds for both groups except for the variance of the latent variable, psychosocial well-being. This is greater for the girls, as can be seen in Fig. 6.4. For all four models, the Coefficient of Determination for physiological status, in this case the same as the Squared Mean Correlation, is between .76 and .77. Figure 6.4 provides the standardised weighted least squares estimates of the final model. The error terms for indicators within each construct are not shown, and can be obtained by subtracting the squared factor loading from a unity ($\theta_\varepsilon = 1-\lambda^2$).

All paths in the model are statistically significant. The negative loading of parental communication on the latent variable 'Psychosocial well-being' indicates an inverse relationship with the other indicators for that latent variable, as does the negative loading of perceived health on physiological status. For instance, good parental communication is related to fewer worries, and good perceived health is related to fewer symptoms.

DISCUSSION

While health is 'the least of their worries', adolescent worries *are* health-related, the topics of adolescent worries as well as the statistics show a relationship with health. Appearance, achievement and emotional upheaval are high rating worries and are related to health outcomes and health behaviour. Appearance is related to eating habits, hygiene, and regular sleeping habits (Sizer, & Whitney, 1997). Achievement in both sport and school requires stamina and concentration. Once again, these are related to proper eating habits and regular sleeping patterns (Pipes,

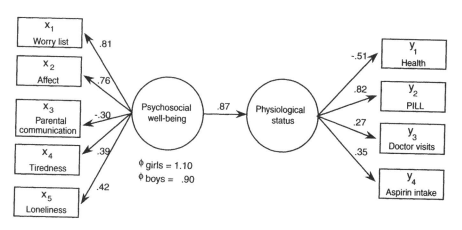

FIG. 6.4   Standardised WLS estimates for the final Model C′ of the relationship between psychosocial well-being and physiological status.

& Trahms, 1993). Emotional upheaval is at the front end of the model. It is not so much a health outcome, but a determinant of health, which in turn influences appearance and achievement. It has been shown that adolescents are often unaware of these interrelationships between certain behaviours, health outcomes, and other desired outcomes (Spruijt-Metz et al., 1994). Health education can be approached by embedding information in the system of worries and interests of the target group and by doing so, activating recognisable motivations for using the knowledge conveyed. By identifying links between typical behaviours, health-related outcomes, and major worries, health education can encourage continuing awareness of relevant cause and effect relationships.

Neither the hierarchy of worries nor the hierarchy of symptoms differs between the genders. The influence of the specific cultural values and norms evident in both of the lists should be noted. The worry list is devoid of issues such as HIV, terrorism, death, and divorce in the family, which figure high on the lists of adolescents in other countries (Carr, & Schmidt, 1994; Hamilton et al., 1988; Kaufman et al., 1993; Klingman, 1998; Orton, 1982). The configuration of cold symptoms in the 'top ten' ranking symptoms is at least partially attributable to the Dutch climate and the fact that the questionnaire was completed in the winter. The high incidence of headache in adolescence has been documented in earlier research (Pothmann, Frankenberg, Müller, Sartory, & Hellmeier, 1994). Possible causes, preventive behaviours and treatments of headaches should be addressed in health education. The substantial disturbance reported by blushing, sensitive teeth, and sleeping problems deserves further research.

The proposed measurement models for the latent variables 'psychosocial well-being' and 'physiological status' fit well for both boys and girls. This means that, taken together, the worry list, negative affectivity, ease of communication with parents, tiredness and loneliness form a meaningful configuration of indicators for one underlying construct labelled here as 'psychosocial well-being'. Also, self-rated health, symptoms, doctors' visits and aspirin consumption can be successfully grouped together as indicators of one underlying construct, labelled here as 'physiological status'. Gender differences were found on six of the nine observed variables, replicating earlier research findings. These gender differences in psychological and physical well-being, repeatedly found in Western populations, could indicate gender-specific, qualitatively different relationships between body and mind, meaning that different constructs contribute in different manners to the explanation of variance in physical distress. The gender differences could also indicate a similar structure and denote differences in degree only, where girls report more, but more of the same. In this case the relationships would be comparable, but girls either experience physical and psychosocial occurrences more intensely, more accurately, tend to report more, or tend to interpret their experiences on a more extreme scale. We find here that the same measurement and structural models fit for both genders with the exception of the variance in psychosocial well-being. It can thus be said that while girls report lower psychosocial well-being in general and a poorer physiological status, the structural relationship between these two constructs is the same for boys and girls.

According to the structural model, 77% of the variance in the physiological status of both boys and girls can be explained by psychosocial well-being, leaving only 23% to be explained by physiological differences, error, and any other sources. In answer to the question of whether worrying is related to health outcomes in adolescence, the answer is 'yes'.

This 'yes' must be annotated. Physiological status is measured here exclusively with self-report, as is psychosocial well-being. For this reason, psychosocial well-being and physiological status might best be labelled *perceived* psychosocial well-being and *perceived* physiological status. However, worries, affect, tiredness and loneliness are purely matters of individual perception, and for many of the physiological complaints studied here, such as headache and nausea, there are no objective measures. When dealing with everyday symptomatology, the difference between objective health and perceived health is therefore difficult if not impossible to discern.

What can be said about the nature of the relationship between psychosocial well-being and physiological status? Bentler (1978) has given a thorough elucidation on the difficulty of drawing causal inferences using structural models. The essence of his explanation is that, although structural modelling has often been referred to as 'causal' modelling, it is a correlational technique, and correlations imply relationships rather than causes. Also, the best fitting model in this study is an equivalent of its mirror image. In other words, flipping the model and allowing physiological status to explain psychosocial well-being delivers a statistically equivalent model to the one chosen here (Hershberger, 1994). The equivalent model, however, implies a very different substantive interpretation of the data. The direction of the model is chosen on the strength of viable theory. Current theory supports psychological precursors of physiological symptoms rather than vice versa. Although the mechanisms by which psychosocial elements affect physiology have not been touched upon here, it is of interest to consider these findings as having bearing upon them. Several mechanisms have been suggested in the literature, including suppression of immunological functions (Wu, & Lam, 1993). The model presented here implies that while the girls report more physical problems because they seem to have more psychosocial problems, similar mechanisms may be at work in both genders.

The conclusion that can be drawn is that psychosocial well-being, including worries, parental communication, negative affectivity, loneliness and tiredness, is strongly related to physiological status in adolescence. Adolescence is a period in which health habits are being formed that will have an effect over the entire life-span (Cobb, 1992). Physical, social, and cognitive changes are taking place which demand considerable adaptation (Kaufman et al., 1993), and the crucial developmental task of the development of the individual's self-image is being negotiated (Erikson, 1963). The physical and social changes can be addressed in conjunction with the elements of psychosocial well-being, such as connecting physical changes with worries about appearance and social changes with parental communication. This can be accomplished while making use of and challenging the high-speed cognitive development that takes place in adolescence. Habits can be encouraged that enhance self-image and are related to positive health outcomes. Relevant health education which addresses the elements of psychosocial well-being adequately can help the adolescent to integrate healthy habits into the growth process, motivate adolescents to keep abreast of new developments in health technology, and contribute to an awareness of relevant causes and effects.

CHAPTER SEVEN

Everyday health and risk behaviours[1]

INTRODUCTION

In this chapter, the data from the survey concerning patterns of everyday health and risk behaviours undertaken during adolescence will be examined. To describe the terrain, the prevalence of various health-related behaviours in relationship to gender and age will be investigated. The focus of the research remains everyday health and risk behaviours, as discussed in Chapter 1. These are common behaviours that influence health, such as eating and sleeping habits. Everyday healthy behaviours are generally approved of, just as everyday risky behaviours are generally discouraged by society. While everyday health and risk behaviours are not ensconced in a stringent moral network, morally laden behaviours such as smoking or unsafe sex are often part of a system of socially negatively qualified behaviour, forcefully condemned by adults, media, institutions, and so forth (Donovan, Jessor, & Costa, 1991). Perhaps because they lack a strong moral framework, everyday healthy behaviours may be easier to ignore, just as everyday risky ones may be more attractive to perform occasionally, in the process of testing one's boundaries and building autonomy during adolescence (Spruijt-Metz, 1998b). While these everyday behaviours are not always the most obvious targets for adolescent health promotion, with the notable exception of eating habits, they make up daily routines that could lay the groundwork for long-term healthy or risky lifestyles. These are the considerations that led to the decision to study everyday behaviours extensively.

---

[1]Parts of this chapter previously appeared as: Spruijt-Metz, D., & Spruijt, R.J. (1996). Alledaags gezondheids- en Risicogedrag van adolescenten [Everyday health and risk behaviour of adolescents]. *Gedrag en Gezondheid, 24*(4), 181–191. Reprinted by permission of Uitgeverij De Tijdstroom.

The viability of the 'lifestyle' approach to prevention and health education will also be explored in this chapter. Lifestyles have been defined as "patterns of (behavioural) choices made from the alternatives that are available to people according to their socio-economic circumstances and to the ease with which they are able to choose certain ones over others", (World Health Organization), 1986, p. 118). It has been suggested that healthy behaviours tend to cluster to form a 'healthy' lifestyle, while risky behaviours tend to cluster into a 'risky' lifestyle (Donovan et al., 1991, 1993). Other authors argue against the study of coherent lifestyles during adolescence (Terre et al., 1992). Some research has pointed towards a multidimensional model of health and risk behaviours that differs for different ethnic-cultural groups (Basen-Engquist, Edmundson, & Parcel, 1996). This means that some behaviours occur together and thus form various behavioural clusters (for instance, an adolescent that smokes tobacco would be more likely to drink alcohol). It also means that behaviours will cluster differently depending upon ethnic-cultural group.

Which of these various approaches is the 'right' one? The advantages of being able to consider healthy behaviours as part of coherent systems of behaviour are immense for health education and promotion. We could then assume that these coherent systems of behaviour form healthy lifestyles, and might also function as buffers against unhealthy lifestyles. This would facilitate theory-driven research and intervention. It also extends the hope that tackling single health or risk behaviours might influence an entire system of related behaviours. Convincing evidence has been provided for the existence of risky adolescent lifestyles. Morally laden problem behaviours have been shown to form a consistently interrelated and coherent group of behaviours that can be explained to a great extent using one theoretical framework (Jessor, 1984, 1991, 1998). However, research on the existence of cohesive healthy adolescent lifestyles has been inconclusive, yielding only moderate relationships between everyday behaviours, which are more difficult to explain within a single theoretical framework (Donovan et al., 1991, 1993; Jessor, 1984, 1991; Terre et al., 1992). Several researchers, such as Kirscht (1983) have expressed doubts concerning the viability of the concept of cohesive healthy adolescent lifestyles, and tend to favour studying health behaviours separately. Studies supporting this point of view show different determinants for different health behaviours and lack of cohesion between them (Basen-Engquist et al., 1996; Cohen, Brownell, & Felix, 1990; Schwarzer, Jerusalem, & Kleine, 1990; Terre et al., 1992).

Whether or not healthy and risky behaviours cluster into lifestyles, they are assumed to influence physical health and psychosocial well-being. It then stands to reason that health and well-being should have a reciprocal relationship with levels of involvement in healthy or risky behaviours. From levels of involvement in health and risk behaviours, we should be able to predict levels of perceived well-being or discomfort. Conversely, feelings of well-being or discomfort should be predictive of the predicating behaviours. Life in general and health interventions in particular would be considerably more straightforward if everyday health-related behaviour had a linear, immediate, and noticeable effect on health. However, research indicates that while risk behaviours are moderately associated with perceived health, healthy behaviours are only weakly related to perceived health (Schwarzer et al., 1990). This relationship is worth further study, if only to establish group and behaviour-specific differences. To understand the role that perceived health may play as a motivation to act on one hand, or as a result of action on the other, we will also look at the relationships between levels of perceived well-being and participation in health-related behaviours.

As we saw in Chapter 6, there is a strong relationship between health, both perceived and objectively ascertained, and measures of psychosocial well-being (Spruijt-Metz, & Spruijt, 1997; Waldron, 1983; Watson, & Pennebaker, 1989; Wu, & Lam, 1993). Much less is known about the relationship between psychosocial well-being and health-related *behaviour* (Terre et al., 1992), with the exception of the research on the influence of peers and parents on health-related behaviour (Janz, & Becker, 1984; Lau, Quadrel, & Hartman, 1990). A strong relationship between psychosocial well-being and health-related behaviour could provide a potentially powerful indirect route to the influence of health, because many elements of psychosocial well-being can be addressed in health intervention programmes for adolescents (Parcel, 1976; Parcel, Simons-Morton, & Kolbe, 1988; Perry, & Kelder, 1992; Sloboda, & David, 1997). By designing health education programmes to include aspects of psychosocial well-being such as communication skills, or dealing with worries and concerns, we might be able to influence everyday health-related behaviours that are otherwise difficult to approach effectively.

In order to fully understand the impact of psychosocial well-being and physical health upon everyday health and risk behaviours, gender and age differences must be studied. Gender differences in perceived health, perceived psychosocial well-being, health behaviour, and risk behaviour have been well documented (Bush, Harkings, Harrington, & Price, 1993; Donovan et al., 1993; Settertobulte, & Kolip, 1997). Girls usually report more symptoms (Pennebaker, 1982; Spruijt-Metz, & Spruijt, 1997), more worries (Kaufman et al., 1993; Klingman, 1998; McGuire et al., 1987; Orton, 1982), more negative affectivity (Watson, & Pennebaker, 1989), and more healthy behaviour in general, with the exception of exercise (Cohen et al., 1990; Terre et al., 1992). Adolescence is a transitional time for health habits, and age is a differential determinant for a number of health-related behaviours during adolescence (Cohen et al., 1990; Terre et al., 1992). As adolescence progresses, health habits, such as attention to diet, tend to deteriorate, and risk behaviours, such as smoking and alcohol consumption, tend to increase (Cohen et al., 1990). Health complaints also increase during adolescence (Spruijt, & Spruijt-Metz, 1994). Appropriate timing may therefore be essential in the planning of health interventions, along with consideration of developmental differences in cognitive abilities and health interests as well as needs. For instance, late adolescents who will soon be making the transition of moving away from home might profit optimally from relatively challenging material about how to make sound dietary choices on a limited budget. Generally speaking, the most opportune moment for effective health education may be when habits (or targeted behaviours) are changing and personal control over health is being tested out (Cohen et al., 1990).

The aims of the analyses presented in this chapter were threefold. The first aim was to examine the prevalences of everyday health and risk behaviours for gender and developmental differences. Considering possible interactions between age and gender, a multivariate approach was taken instead of a univariate one (Terre et al., 1992). The second aim was to study the predictive value of psychosocial well-being and perceived physical health for everyday health behaviours and risk behaviours. In keeping with the reciprocal relationships between well-being and behaviour as found in Chapter 6, the direction of prediction must be regarded as a theoretical choice. Because gender and development are known to be related to health behaviour, psychosocial well-being, and perceived physical health, analyses were done differentially for early adolescent girls, early adolescent boys, late adolescent girls, and late adolescent boys. The third aim of the study was to compare the viability of the lifestyle approach for the study of everyday health and risk behaviours to the validity of the single behaviour approach. To do this, the association between the various health behaviours and risk behaviours was examined.

METHODS AND MATERIALS

Subjects

The sample and procedure are described in detail in the previous chapter.

Dependent variables: Health and risk behaviours

The inventories of everyday health and risk behaviours were developed specifically for the present research using preliminary unstructured interviews followed by open questionnaires and focus group interviews (Chapters 4 and 5). The resulting 18 items (see Table 7.3) show the everyday behaviours which the target group found important and understood as healthy or risky. Most of the health behaviours were 'mirrored' in risk behaviours, such as healthy diet vs. poor diet. Eating a lot of sweets was consistently experienced as a risk behaviour with its own status, apart from poor dietary habits, and was added to the list of risk behaviours accordingly. The subjects were asked to what extent they performed each of the behaviours to stay healthy. The frequency with which each behaviour is carried out was measured on a five-point scale (1 = never to 5 = often).

While there was only a modest association between everyday health behaviours (Cronbach's alpha = .55), the risk behaviour items form a fairly homogeneous scale (Cronbach's alpha = .71). These reliability scores remained consistent after transformation to correct for skewed distributions. The stronger covariation of risk behaviours as opposed to the relatively loose relationships between health behaviours has been ascertained in earlier studies (Dohrenwend, & Shrout, 1985; Donovan et al., 1991, 1993).

Predictors: Perceived psychosocial well-being and perceived physical health

In Chapter 6, we saw that our indicators of perceived psychosocial well-being and perceived physical health fit the data. Composite factor scores for psychosocial well-being and physiological status were generated in SPSS using factor loadings. A high score on psychosocial well-being indicates more worries, more loneliness, more tiredness, a higher score on negative affect, and poorer communication with parents. A high score on physiological status indicates more physical complaints, poorer perceived health, more frequent visits to the doctor, and more aspirin use.

Demographic variables: Gender and developmental stage

Questions about gender and age were posed on the first page of the questionnaire. To examine the influence of age on health and on risk behaviours, the subjects are grouped into two developmental stages: early adolescence (up to 14 years of age), and late adolescence (15 years of age and up) (Cobb, 1998).

Analyses

To examine gender and developmental differences on the individual health behaviours, on the individual risk behaviours, on the composite scores of health and risk behaviours, and on the factor scores for psychosocial well-being and physiological status, four MANOVAs were carried out.

Box 7.1: Methods box: Using Multivariate Analysis of Variance (MANOVA)

After the strong defence I gave of using Structural Modelling in Chapter 6, you might ask why I am using MANOVA in Chapter 7. Good question. If you remember from the last chapter, in order to use Structural Modelling, a measurement model has to be constructed and it has to fit the data. For the data analysed in this chapter, that meant that the indicators for health behaviour and risk behaviour had to form viable factors. As will be discussed later on, health behaviours and risk behaviours didn't really form coherent latent variables. As you read through this chapter, you will find that the data do not support 'healthy' lifestyles versus 'unhealthy' lifestyles. Things are more complex. Some behaviours do seem to cluster, but the clusters are not always theoretically logical, other behaviours stand

Box 7.1 continued

Box 7.1: Methods box: Using Multivariate Analysis of Variance (MANOVA) (continued)

alone. Without a fitting measurement model for theoretically sound latent variables, Structural Equation Modelling won't work.

The data to be analysed for this chapter includes more than two groups (early adolescent girls and boys, late adolescent girls and boys). So *t*-tests are out of the question because there are more than two groups. The data also include more than one dependent variable. So you could conceivably use a series of ANOVAs, but this would lead to multiple testing which increases your chance of Type I error. In this situation, MANOVA is indicated.

MANOVA tests whether mean differences among groups on a combination of dependent variables are likely to have occurred by chance. It has some advantages and some disadvantages.

Advantages of doing a single MANOVA instead of a series of ANOVA:
(1) Protection against the inflated Type I error that goes along with multiple testing.
(2) MANOVA creates a new dependent variable from the set of original dependent variables that maximises group differences. For this and other reasons, MANOVA might be more powerful than ANOVA. Sometimes.

Disadvantages of using MANOVA:
(1) Partially because MANOVA creates that new DV, your results can be very hard to interpret. It can be really difficult to understand the relationships between single independent and dependent variables (Tabachnick, & Fidell, 1996). So you might end out doing a series of ANOVAs after all is said and done.
(2) The temptation to include highly correlated dependent variables is great because MANOVA makes inclusion of multiple dependent variables so easy. This encourages researchers to add them all rather than go through the painful process of checking for correlations, weeding out multiple measures, and choosing the theoretically important variables beforehand.
(3) Furthermore, MANOVA is sensitive to missing data and unequal sample sizes. There are stringent requirements as to the number of cases as opposed to the number of dependent variables (more cases than dependent variables in every cell).

In short, one should **proceed with caution** when using this data analytical technique.

To compare health and risk behaviour priorities of early and late adolescent girls and boys, comparability of the order of mean scores on the individual health and risk behaviour items were computed using Spearman's rank correlation coefficient.

Hierarchical regression analyses were carried out to determine the amount of independent variation in the composite health and risk behaviour scores accounted for by gender, stage, psychosocial well-being and physiological status, in that order. The additional reciprocal effects of health and risk behaviour were examined by entering one to the regression equation of the other as the last step. These hierarchical regression analyses were repeated for the separate health and risk behaviours.

RESULTS

From the 416 subjects that participated in the study, those outside the age range of 12 to 17 years were omitted from the analysis to obtain a more homogeneous age group. Eight multivariate outlying cases, identified using Mahalanobis distance at an alpha = .01 cut-off level, were also deleted from the analysis (Stevens, 1992). No univariate outlying cases were detected after square root transformations of the risk behaviour measurements for oral and general hygiene. Student's t-tests between groups with and without missing values on the dependent and independent variables did not show systematic differences. Missing values were distributed equally over gender and stage groups, and discriminant analysis using the variables included in this study showed a 50–50 chance of predicting cases with missing values, suggesting that the missing values were distributed randomly over the sample and could be deleted (Tabachnick, & Fidell, 1996). The effective sample size was 363 (111 early adolescent girls, 77 late adolescent girls, 104 early adolescent boys, and 71 late adolescent boys).

Gender and stage differences

Four MANOVAs were carried out to examine gender and stage differences in health behaviours, risk behaviours, the composite scores for health and for risk behaviours, and the predictor factors (psychosocial well-being and physiological status). In this case, to insure against the possibility of inflated Type I errors due to deviations from univariate normality and the perils of multiple testing, a very stringent alpha level ($\alpha = .001$) was employed (Stevens, 1992) .

Table 7.1 shows the results of the multivariate F-tests from the four MANOVAs using Wilks' criterion.

Main effects of gender and stage were found on all the variables in the multivariate analyses. No interaction effects were found between gender and stage. The effect of gender was consistently larger than the effect of stage, except on risk behaviour, where both effects were moderate.

Descriptive statistics and the results of the univariate F-tests from the MANOVAs on the health behaviour composite score, risk behaviour composite score, psychosocial well-being and physiological status are presented in Table 7.2.

Girls reported more health behaviours, but did not report fewer risk behaviours. Girls reported poorer psychosocial well-being, and the substantial effect of gender on perceived physiological status shows that the boys reported feeling a great deal better than the girls did. The small but consistent effect of stage on all variables shows late adolescents undertook fewer healthy behaviours, more risky behaviours, and reported poorer health and well-being.

Descriptive statistics and the results of the univariate F-tests from the MANOVAs on each of the health and risk behaviours are presented in Table 7.3.

TABLE 7.1

Results of the multivariate *F*-tests from MANOVA's on health behaviours, risk behaviours, the composite scores for health and risk behaviours, and the predictor factors (psychosocial well-being and physiological status) by gender and age group

Variable	*F*	df	η^{2a}
Health behaviours			
Main effect sex	7.98*	9, 351	.10
Main effect age	4.13*	9, 351	.10
Interaction sex/age	.99	9, 351	—
Risk behaviours			
Main effect sex	4.80*	9, 351	.11
Main effect age	4.06*	9, 351	.09
Interaction sex/age	.99	9, 351	—
Composite scores			
Main effect sex	17.85*	2, 358	.09
Main effect age	10.39*	2, 358	.05
Interaction sex/age	.31	2, 358	—
Predictor factors			
Main effect sex	30.85*	2, 358	.14
Main effect age	8.84*	2, 358	.05
Interaction sex/age	.70	2, 358	—

$^a\eta^2$: .01 = small effect, .06 = medium effect, .14 = large effect (adapted from Cohen, 1988).

*p <.001.

TABLE 7.2

Descriptive statistics and univariate *F*-tests from MANOVAs on the composite scores for health and for risk behaviour, and for the predictor factors (psychosocial well-being and physiological status) by gender and age group

	Girls (n=188)		Boys (n=175)		Effect Gender		Effect Stage	
	12–14 years	15–17 years	12–14 yrs.	15–17 years				
Variable	$\bar{X}$ (SD)	$\bar{X}$ (SD)	$\bar{X}$ (SD)	$\bar{X}$ (SD)	F^a	η^{2b}	F^a	η^{2b}
Composite scores								
Health behaviour composite	3.97(.36)	3.82(.40)	3.77(.47)	3.55(.47)	27.05*	.07	16.77*	.05
Risk behaviour composite	2.12(.52)	2.34(52)	2.10(.65)	2.34(.61)	.04	–	13.63*	.04
Predictor factors^c								
Psychosocial well-being	.08(1.05)	.46(.84)	-.36(.91)	-.12(1.02)	23.94*	.06	9.12*	.03
Physiological status	.16(.97)	.66(1.03)	-.49(.75)	-.22(.92)	60.19*	.14	16.25*	.04

^{a}df for univariate tests: 1, 359.

$^b\eta^2$: .01 = small effect, .06 = medium effect, .14 = large effect.

^{c} Negative and low scores indicate fewer physical complaints and fewer psychosocial hassles. High scores on physiological status and psychosocial well-being indicate more complaints and lower degree of well-being, respectively.

* p <.001.

TABLE 7.3

Descriptive statistics and univariate F-tests from MANOVAs on the individual health behaviours and risk behaviours by gender and age group

| Variable | Girls (n=188) | | Boys (n=175) | | Effect Gender | | Effect Stage | |
	12–14 years X̄(SD)	15–17 years X̄(SD)	12–14 yrs. X̄(SD)	15–17 years X̄(SD)	F^a	η^{2b}	F^a	η^{2b}
Health behaviours								
Good hygiene	4.77(.49)	4.83(.41)	4.63(.58)	4.62(.64)	9.20	—	.30	—
Good oral hygiene	4.73(.50)	4.83(.41)	4.57(.65)	4.45(.73)	17.66*	.05	.03	—
Warm clothing	4.44(.75)	4.27(.82)	4.35(.79)	4.07(.93)	2.43	—	6.86	—
Enough sports	4.27(.80)	3.90(1.01)	4.58(.77)	4.09(1.07)	7.96	—	19.62*	.05
Careful in traffic	4.15(.92)	4.14(.82)	3.82(1.11)	3.63(1.29)	13.47*	.04	.79	—
Enough sleep	4.17(.89)	3.83(.90)	3.82(1.01)	3.47(1.07)	13.18*	.04	11.93*	.03
Healthy diet	3.47(.88)	3.09(1.15)	3.33(1.01)	3.31(1.10)	.01	—	3.48	—
Talk about problems	3.54(1.07)	3.43(1.18)	2.90(1.26)	2.70(1.12)	30.95*	.08	1.69	—
Take vitamins	2.18(1.36)	2.04(1.40)	1.90(1.24)	1.58(1.01)	7.11	—	2.75	—
Risk behaviours								
Eat a lot of sweets	3.03(1.23)	3.34(1.14)	2.74(1.21)	2.93(1.18)	7.21	—	3.90	—
Poor diet	2.53(.77)	3.01(.99)	2.42(1.01)	2.86(.96)	1.73	—	21.27*	.06
Too little sleep	2.50(.96)	2.86(1.05)	2.41(1.21)	2.89(1.10)	.14	—	12.61*	.03
Not talk about problems	2.12(1.06)	2.44(1.16)	2.00(1.07)	2.47(1.22)	.27	—	10.79*	.03
No warm clothing	1.97(.97)	2.20(.95)	1.98(1.12)	2.06(.94)	.25	—	1.99	—
Not enough sports	1.95(1.18)	2.22(1.20)	1.67(1.08)	2.00(1.12)	4.41	—	6.00*	.02
Fool around in traffic	1.67(.77)	1.65(.82)	2.13(1.24)	2.18(1.16)	21.02*	.06	.03	—
Poor oral hygiene	1.28(.32)	1.27(.37)	1.29(.36)	1.30(.35)	.28	—	.00	—
Poor hygiene	1.22(.28)	1.22(.31)	1.18(.35)	1.31(.35)	4.46	—	.20	—
Total N = 363	n = 111	n = 77	n = 104	n = 71				

[a]df for univariate tests: 1, 359.

[b]η^2: .01 = small effect, .06 = medium effect, .14 = large effect.

* $p < .001$.

Gender had more significant effects on health behaviours than did stage. The girls reported better oral hygiene, more caution in traffic, more sleep, and more frequent discussion of their problems. Stage differences in health behaviours were represented by reports of more hours of sleep and more exercise by the early adolescents. On the risk behaviours, there were more significant effects of stage than of gender. The only significant gender difference showed the boys taking more risks in traffic. Stage differences showed poorer eating habits, later bedtimes, less communications about problems, and less sports activities in late adolescence. As can be seen by these results, reports on 'mirror image' health and risk behaviours are not always related. For instance, while late adolescents score higher than early adolescents do on risky diet, they do not score lower on healthy diet, as might be expected.

The largest effect of gender was on talking about one's problems, where both early and late adolescent girls far outdid the boys. The largest effect of stage was on poor eating habits. Diet seemed to deteriorate for both boys and girls in late adolescence.

The health and risk behaviours in Table 7.3 are ranked in order of importance according to the entire sample. However, the differences in hierarchies of health and risk behaviours suggest that gender and stage differences may not only be a question of degree, but also one of structure, priorities and interests. Spearman's rank correlation coefficient (r_S) was significant ($p < .001$) for the ranking of *health* behaviours by early and late adolescent boys ($r_S = .97$), but nor for the ranking of *risk* behaviours for the same groups ($r_S = .70, p > .02$). Spearman's rank correlation coefficient was significant for the ranking of *risk* behaviours by early and late adolescent girls ($r_S = .97$), but not for the ranking of *health* behaviours for the same groups ($r_S = .70, p > .02$). The rest of the comparisons between girls and boys for both stages and both categories of behaviour were not significant, the lowest r_S being between the ranking of health behaviours by early adolescent boys and late adolescent girls ($r_S = .14, p > .34$).

Predicting health and risk behaviours

Results of the hierarchical regression analyses for the composite scores on health and risk behaviours are presented in Table 7.4.

Gender, stage, and (negative) psychosocial well-being explained a significant, albeit not large, amount of the variance in health behaviour. Stage and (negative) psychosocial well-being alone explained 23% of the variance in risk behaviour, and the link between (negative) psychosocial well-being and risk behaviours was the strongest in the analyses. Gender does not contribute to the explanation of variance in risk behaviours. Consistent with the findings of Donovan et al. (1991) and other researchers, the variance explained in health behaviour by risk behaviour and vice versa showed a systematic, if modest, relationship between the two composite scores. Salient here is that perceived physiological status did not contribute significantly to either equation. This was also the case when physiological status was entered into the equation before psychosocial well-being. In other words, perceived health did not influence behaviour.

Results of the hierarchical multiple regression analyses on the scores for the individual health and risk behaviours are shown in Table 7.5.

The amount of explained variance in the individual health and risk behaviour scores was consistently lower than for the composite scores. The largest amount of explained variance was for both healthy and risky sleeping habits, although the prediction was not always similar for 'mirrored' behaviours, nor did the same predictors always contribute significantly to the equation of 'mirrored' behaviours. The only behaviour for which a significant amount of variance could not be explained by the variables considered here was 'taking vitamins', most likely because there was not much variance to explain, and the mean score was low (see Table 7.3). The individual analyses upheld the predictive values of the four gender

TABLE 7.4

Hierarchical multiple regression analyses on composite health and risk behaviour composite scores

Predictor	B	β	R^2 change		
Dependent variable: Health behaviour composite					
Gender	−.27	−.31	.07*		
Stage	−.09	−.10	.04*	Intercept	5.04
Psychosocial well-being	.01	.01	.05*	R^2	.31*
Physiological status	−.05	−.11	.01	Adjusted R^2	.30
Risk behaviour composite	−.33	−.43	.14*	R	.56*
Dependent variable: Risk behaviour composite					
Gender	−.04	−.04	.00		
Stage	.07	.06	.04*	Intercept	4.15
Psychosocial well-being	.22	.38	.19*	R^2	.36*
Physiological status	−.03	−.05	.00	Adjusted R^2	.35
Health behaviour composite	−.52	−.40	.13*	R	.60*

Significance of R^2 change was determined by the general F-test for an increment.

High scores on psychosocial well-being and physiological status indicate *more* complaints. Positive relationships with either variable means that higher scores on a health or risk behaviour are associated with lowered psychosocial well-being and poorer physiological status. Negative relationships mean that high scores on health or risk behaviour is associated with greater psychosocial well-being and better physiological status.

*$p < .001$.

differences found in health behaviours and the one found on risk behaviours in the MANOVAs. The effect of stage differences found in the MANOVAs for 'not enough sports' was apparently not large enough to contribute significantly to the regression equation, leaving significant contributions of stage for two health behaviours and three risk behaviours. Of course, the most consistent predictor for health behaviour was lack of involvement in risk behaviours, and vice versa, while all significant mutual contributions were nonetheless small. Health behaviours buffered risk behaviours, but not to a great extent. This weak relationship elucidates the fact that, regardless of the buffering effects, while girls reported more health behaviours, they did not report fewer risk behaviours (Tables 7.2 and 7.3). Negative psychosocial well-being contributed significantly to all but two of the equations for risk behaviours, and also made the two largest contributions to any of the equations in the analyses (for 'too little sleep' and 'not talking about problems'). Once again, physiological status did not contribute significantly to any of the equations, which was also the case when the order of entry into the equations was changed. Table 7.6 provides correlations which, together with the descriptive statistics in Tables 7.2 and 7.3, aid in interpreting the relationships found in the regression analyses.

TABLE 7.5

Hierarchical multiple regression analyses on individual health and risk behaviours

Predictors	Gender R^2 ch.	Stage R^2 ch.	Psychosocial well-being R^2 ch.	Physiological status R^2 ch.	Risk composite R^2 ch.	Total R^2
Dependent variable: Health behaviours						
Good hygiene	.025	.001	.009	.001	.039*	.08*
Good oral hygiene	.047*	.000	.012	.000	.072*	.13*
Warm clothing	.007	.019	.028*	.001	.041*	.10*
Enough sports	.021	.051*	.042*	.020	.008	.14*
Careful in traffic	.036*	.002	.026	.000	.040*	.10*
Enough sleep	.034*	.031*	.067*	.004	.095*	.23*
Healthy diet	.000	.010	.018	.007	.051*	.09*
Talk about problems	.079*	.004	.001	.009	.016	.11*
Take vitamins	.019	.008	.001	.004	.007	.04

Predictors	Gender R^2 ch.	Stage R^2 ch.	Psychosocial well-being R^2 ch.	Physiological status R^2 ch.	Health composite R^2 ch.	Total R^2
Dependent variable: Risk behaviours						
Eat a lot of sweets	.020	.011	.067*	.001	.034*	.13*
Poor diet	.115	.056*	.043*	.000	.024	.13*
Too little sleep	.001	.034*	.143*	.001	.086*	.26*
Not talk about problems	.001	.030*	.122*	.001	.031*	.18*
No warm clothing	.001	.001	.100*	.001	.029*	.13*
Not enough sports	.012	.016	.030*	.000	.035*	.09*
Fool around in traffic	.055*	.000	.023	.003	.037*	.12*
Poor oral hygiene	.001	.000	.030*	.003	.058*	.09*
Poor hygiene	.013	.001	.015	.001	.040*	.07*

*$p < .001$.

Let us have a look at the correlations and see how they can help us interpret the findings. For instance, the score of the health behaviour for which the most variance is explained also has the highest negative correlation with risk behaviour. Using Tables 7.2, 7.3 and 7.6 we see that this behaviour, 'getting enough sleep', is related to being a girl, being an early adolescent, experiencing satisfactory psychosocial well-being, and abstaining from risk behaviours in general. The risk behaviour 'too little sleep' has the highest negative correlation with health behaviour. While gender does not play a role in the prediction here, stage and psychosocial well-being do. The older subjects who score lower on psychosocial well-being and on participation in health behaviours get less sleep. Gender differences are the only predictor for the health behaviour 'talking about problems'. The girls are more apt to talk about their problems. However, for prediction of the risk behaviour 'not talking about problems', gender differences are not relevant. Late adolescents who score lower on psychosocial well-being and on participation in health behaviours are less likely to talk about their problems.

TABLE 7.6

Correlations of health and risk behaviours with psychosocial well-being, physiological status, and the health and risk behaviour composite scores

	Psychosocial well-being	Physiological status	Behaviour composite
Health behaviours			
Good hygiene	−.05	−.00	−.21*
Good oral hygiene	−.06	.02	−.29*
Warm clothing	−.16*	−.10	−.28*
Enough sports	−.26*	−.30*	−.22*
Careful in traffic	−.12	−.01	−.25*
Enough sleep	−.23*	−.13*	−.42*
Healthy diet	−.14*	−.15*	−.28*
Talk about problems	.09	.03	−.11
Take vitamins	.05	.09	−.08
Health composite score	−.19*	−.12*	−.47*
Risk behaviours			
Eat a lot of sweets	.30*	.22*	−.22*
Poor diet	.25*	.16*	−.22*
Too little sleep	.39*	.23*	−.39*
Not talk about problems	.36*	.23*	−.28*
No warm clothing	.32*	.14*	−.24*
Not enough sports	.21*	.15*	−.21*
Fool around in traffic	.09	−.06	−.27*
Poor oral hygiene	.16*	.02	−.27*
Poor hygiene	.09	.03	−.25*
Risk composite score	.44*	.23*	−.47*

High scores on psychosocial well-being and physiological status indicate *more* complaints. Positive correlation with either variable means that higher scores on a health or risk behaviour are related to lowered psychosocial well-being and poorer physiological status.
$*p < .01$.

DISCUSSION

These results support the concept of a cohesive *risky* adolescent lifestyle. If an adolescent participates in one risky behaviour, it is probable that he or she will participate in other risky behaviours. Risk behaviours form a cohesive scale, and are fairly consistently related to negative psychosocial well-being and infrequent healthy behaviours. This suggests that risky adolescent lifestyles could be buffered by effective health education including training in health behaviour and psychosocial skills.

The evidence for a cohesive adolescent *healthy* lifestyle is less convincing. If an adolescent undertakes one healthy behaviour, it is not necessarily probable that he or she will undertake others. The prediction of the composite score for health behaviours is comparable to that of the composite score for risk behaviours, and better than that for the individual behaviours. This, along with the theoretical advantages of being able to refer to a complex of behaviours as a 'healthy lifestyle', makes it tempting to continue using composite health behaviour measures. However, the relationship between healthy behaviours is not strong, Cronbach's alpha is low and no interpretable and reliable pattern emerged in preliminary factor analyses. In using a composite measure for groups of weakly correlated health behaviours to represent the concept of a healthy lifestyle, we are predicting something that we cannot measure well (and therefore might not exist). The lack of cohesion between healthy behaviours is confirmed when the individual behaviours are examined. No consistent combination of predictors emerges. No two health behaviours are alike, which leads to the conclusion that health behaviours are best approached separately. There is, however, a reciprocal negative relationship between two-thirds of the individual health behaviours studied here and risk behaviour in general. Therefore, while we cannot equitably refer to an overall healthy lifestyle, participating in healthy behaviours may be said to hinder participation in risky ones to some degree.

A dominant conceptual framework in the field (and the one in which this study is placed), assumes that health behaviour and risk behaviour represent two distinct categories of behaviour. Although the use of the separate categories has an important heuristic value and is embedded in our way of judging actions, no empirical support was found here for this conceptual framework. Behaviours that are risky are often related to behaviours that are healthy, and healthy behaviours are often unrelated to one another. Instead of relying solely upon these separate categories, it might make sense to work within a loosely structured concept of health-related behaviours, in which both categories are subsumed.

Negative psychosocial well-being, encompassing worrying, negative affect, being tired, feeling lonely, and unsatisfactory communications with parents, was predictive for seven out of nine risk behaviours, and positive psychosocial well-being predicted three of the health behaviours. Psychosocial well-being is thus a promising area for further research in health and risk behaviour during adolescence, including examination of the extent to which the individual elements can be mediated and how these can best be approached in health promotion programmes for adolescents.

A striking result is that perceived physical health is not at all related to health behaviour or risk behaviour. Logically, it could be expected that if poor physical health is experienced, action might be taken, or if many health-risks are taken, poor health might be experienced. However, the data indicate that we, as health educators, cannot rely upon a direct response to perceived physical problems, and that there is a hiatus in the perception of cause and effect along these lines. This lack of connection between experienced health and actual behaviour means that a direct approach to health education, in which the links between behaviour and health are elucidated, will not meet with much recognition in the experiential world of the adolescent.

It seems that gender differences might also best be studied at the level of individual behaviour. Girls report more health behaviour in general, but the effect is differential and pertains to less than half of the health behaviours studied here. Gender differences were found on only one of the risk behaviours: 'fooling around in traffic'. For the Dutch population of this age group, this refers to bicycling, riding a moped, and walking. Because traffic safety of our youth is a major concern internationally (World Health Organization, 1998), the extent to which boys who fool around in traffic (on their bikes or otherwise) will do so later behind the wheel deserves further study.

Developmental differences also lend themselves to more detailed study at the level of individual behaviours. A definite pattern emerges, showing late adolescents to be more likely to undertake risky everyday health behaviours. This emphasises the desirability of timing health education interventions to match developmental changes in everyday behaviours. The lack of interaction between the effects of gender and stage suggests that, while the multivariate approach inevitably offers more detailed information, separate study of their effects is justified.

Although the consistent pattern of results under stringent criteria suggests that the findings are valid, this study has the same potential problems inherent in any study of self-reported behaviour. Behavioural measurements and objective measures of symptoms or health would add strength to the design and improve validity.

The limitations of the population studied here have been discussed in Chapter 6. Of interest, then, is not only the degree to which these findings might generalise to similar adolescent populations, but the sort of differences that might be found between different (cultural) groups, to what these differences might be attributed, and their implications for health education and promotion.

The results of this study support the existence of *risky* adolescent lifestyles. However, these results do *not* support the concept of coherent *healthy* lifestyles during adolescence. This means that one *risk* behaviour will most likely lead to other risk behaviours and fewer health behaviours, but that one *health* behaviour will *not* necessarily lead to other health behaviours, although health behaviours generally buffer risk behaviours. Risk behaviours thus seem more malleable, because if a single behaviour can be influenced or changed, several others will most likely follow suit. On the other hand, health behaviours, while they can be promoted effectively, must be approached separately. This is admittedly more work. But the results of this and other studies show that participating in some healthy behaviours may effectively inhibit participation in risky behaviours. These findings have important implications for the further study of health and risk behaviours. The study presented in this book focused almost exclusively on healthy behaviours, with health promotion in mind. Much of the literature on adolescent health has focused almost exclusively on risky behaviours, with prevention in mind. The evidence presented here points towards a more integrated approach, one that studies both healthy and risky behaviours and aims towards a balanced amalgamation of active promotion and prevention.

CHAPTER EIGHT

Personal incentives as determinants of adolescent health behaviour: The meaning of behaviour[1]

INTRODUCTION

This third phase of the research had been undertaken with five goals in mind: (1) to appraise current knowledge about health in the adolescent population, (2) to inventory perceived health and take stock of the health complaints of the group, (3) to assess health and risk behaviours adolescents undertake, (4) to explore the feasibility of reaching different cultural groups with the same material, and (5) to uncover possible determinants of health and risk behaviour. All but the last one have been addressed in the previous chapters. In this chapter, the predictive power of salient meanings of everyday health and risk behaviours will be explored.

The hypothesis that personal, intrinsic meanings of behaviour are major determinants of everyday health and risk behaviour in adolescence had emerged from the focus group interviews and from the literature. Of the several models reviewed in Chapter 3, Tappe's model of Personal Investment (1992) emerged as one of the most interesting. The model was designed to explain adolescent health-related behaviour maximally as well as to provide a comprehensive theoretical framework for the development of effective health education for adolescents. The advantages of this meshing of theory, research, and intervention have been widely recognised (Glanz et al., 1990, 1997; Hochbaum et al., 1992). The model of Personal Investment is an integrative, ecological model. Both personal aspects of behaviour and environmental factors that influence behaviour are taken into

---

[1]Parts of this chapter previously appeared as: Spruijt-Metz, D. (1995). Personal incentives as determinants of adolescent health behavior: The meaning of behavior. *Health Education and Research: Theory and Practice, 10*(3), 355–364. Reprinted by permission of Oxford University Press.

account. This is in congruence with criteria set by frameworks such as PRECEDE (Green, & Kreuter, 1991), the Problem Behaviour theory (Jessor, 1984), and the Social Learning theory (Bandura, 1977b) and as is advocated by many researchers (Diekstra, & Methorst, 1986; Gochman, 1988; Hurrelmann, 1990; Jessor, 1993, 1998; Perry, & Kelder, 1992).

As we learned in Chapter 3, many of the models prevailing in adult health behaviour research assume a basically rational person: one who makes reasonable choices in an autonomous fashion according to available information (Beauchamp, & Childress, 1989). This assumption, however, does not appear to hold consistently for adolescent populations (Brown et al., 1991; Kirscht, 1988). A major strength of the model of Personal Investment is the attempt made to incorporate more emotional aspects of adolescent health behaviour. Tappe bases her model on Maehr and Braskamp's theory of Personal Investment (Maehr, & Braskamp, 1986), which has several commonalties with the revised version of the Protection Motivation theory (Maddux, & Rogers, 1983). Her theory puts forth the subjective meaning of behaviour as the critical determinant of engagement in that behaviour. This central construct is referred to as personal investment meaning, and is conceived of as comprising six interrelated (sub)constructs: sense of self-perceptions, personal incentives, perceived barriers, perceived options, perceived situational opportunities, and perceived situational climate.

One criticism of the model of Personal Investment is that it fails to fully incorporate the role of emotions in behaviour due to an inadequate representation of the influence of the adolescents' emotional world (Tappe, 1992). It has been suggested that a number of the constructs and sub-constructs of the model need to be carefully reanalysed and tested (Glanz et al., 1990).

The emotional elements of behaviour are covered in the model predominantly by the personal incentives construct. Personal incentives are defined as the reasons why adolescents engage in a given health-related behaviour. The incentives are seen to be both intrinsic and extrinsic. In Chapter 5, it seemed that the personal, intrinsic meanings with which adolescents imbue behaviours emerged as more influential for behaviour than any extrinsic incentive. The meanings of behaviour as I would like to define them here are similar to the sets of anticipated outcomes or expectancies advocated by Stacy et al. (1994), except for their purely intrinsic character. While these meanings are often related to extrinsic events, they are intrinsic in that the incentives have to do purely with personal feelings and fantasies. The meaning with which behaviour is imbued is often disassociated from available knowledge and information. For instance, eating sweets may be disassociated from the knowledge that it is unhealthy, bad for one's teeth, fattening, and so forth, and come to represent a way of dealing with frustration, anger, authority, or stress. A few examples from the focus groups (Chapter 5, this book) are revealing:

> Even though I know that smoking is very unhealthy, and I think it is really stupid to do, when I'm angry at my mother, I just HAVE to smoke!

Or: If I don't break the rules every once in a while (and basically do something rather dangerous), then I'm just not alive, not free.

Here we examine the intrinsic aspects of personal incentives are independently from the extrinsic aspects. The predictive values of personal meanings within three realms of everyday behaviour are investigated. These are eating habits at lunch, eating habits after school, and sleeping habits.

METHODS AND MATERIALS

Subjects and procedure

The sample and procedure are described in detail in Chapter 6.

Criterion variables

Three behaviour domains were examined: sleeping habits, eating habits at lunch, and eating habits after school. Sleeping habits were represented by the subjects' perceptions of their own bedtimes during the week. They could choose between (1) early, (2) on time, and (3) late. Lunch habits were assessed so as to place the students into one of three groups: (1) the frequent abstainers, (2) the basically healthy eaters (sandwiches, fruit, and vegetables), and (3) the junk food group (sweets and snack foods such as French fries). The same procedures were followed to appraise eating habits after school.

Predictor variables

Ten items representing the possible meaning of sleeping behaviour, eight items for eating habits at lunch, and seven items for eating habits after school were generated based on data from the focus group interviews (see Tables 8.1, 8.2, and 8.3). For each behaviour, the participants chose the section of the questionnaire that corresponded to his or her own behaviour. If the subject went to be very early, he or she answered the questions on one page, while those who went to bed at a regular time or very late were instructed to go on to pages with the heading corresponding to their own behaviour. Items were of necessity worded differently for each behaviour to avoid nonsense items, and in this way often represented continuums. For instance, for those go to bed early, the cosiness continuum was represented by: 'I go to bed early because it is not pleasant at home in the evenings', while for those who go to bed late, it was represented by 'I stay up late because it is so cosy at home in the living room with everyone else'. Cosiness is the motivation for one behaviour, while lack of cosiness is the motivation for the other. The items were scored on a Likert scale ranging from 1 (totally agree) to 5 (totally disagree). Negatively formulated items were recoded where appropriate.

Analysis

The contribution of the meaning of behaviour to the prediction of that behaviour was studied using stepwise discriminant function analyses (Wilks's method). Analyses were carried out for each of the three behavioural domains: sleeping habits, eating habits at lunch, and eating habits after school. For each domain, the meaning of behaviour was used as a predictor of membership in three groups.

RESULTS

The sample size (over 20 in each group represented in the discriminant analyses) ensured robustness against any violations of the assumption of multivariate normality (Klecka, 1980; Tabachnick, & Fidell, 1996). To take unequal group membership into account, adjustments were made for prior probabilities (Klecka, 1980). This adjustment, along with the sample size, helped to secure robustness with respect to the heterogeneity of variance-covariance matrices found in all three analyses (Lachenbruch, 1975).

Sleeping habits

The first discriminant analysis predicted membership in three groups representing different sleeping habits. The classification procedure included seven items representing the meaning of the behaviours. Of the original sample of 416 subjects,

---

Box 8.1: A word on Discriminant Analysis

As Tabachnik and Fidell (1996) note, Discriminant Analysis is basically MANOVA in the reverse. The question you ask in MANOVA is: "Does group membership produce reliable and real differences on the scores of a dependent variable?" You are usually asking if membership in the treatment group produces differences in outcome scores (or if being an early or late adolescent boy or a girl produces differences in behaviour). Discriminant Analysis asks if differences in scores on (a combination of) variables can predict group membership. The question you might ask Discriminant Analysis is: "If we only know a subject's score on a particular dependent variable, will that allow us to predict whether the subject was in the treatment group or the control group accurately?" In the case of the research presented here, the question might be phrased as follows: "Let's say we only know the scores on the meaning of a particular behaviour. Can we predict from those scores alone whether or not that behaviour was actually engaged in?" This can provide very handy information, especially if you are guessing that in the future, it will be easier to get the scores used to predict behaviour than to measure the subjects' actual behaviour. A variable that allows you to tell groups apart has good powers of discrimination (between groups)—hence the name of the analytic technique. A variable that can discriminate between subjects grouped by the behaviours they undertake can be said to be a predictor of that behaviour.

377 were included in the analysis and 39 were excluded owing to missing data. Actual group membership was: go to bed early ($n = 28$, 7%), go to bed on time ($n = 270$, 72%), and go to bed too late ($n = 79$, 21%). Missing cases were randomly spread throughout the groups.

Two discriminant functions were calculated, with a combined $\chi^2 (14) = 159.06$, $p < .001$. After removal of the first function, the second function was not significant $\chi^2 (6) = 11.94$, $p = .06$. The two discriminant functions accounted for 94% and 6% of the between-group variability. Figure 8.1 shows that the first discriminant function (interpreted as the social function) separates the group that goes to bed late from the on time group, with the early group close to the on time group, while the second function (interpreted as the emotional function) discriminates somewhat between the early group and the other two groups.

A loading matrix of correlations between predictor variables and discriminant functions, as seen in Table 8.1, suggests that the amount of sleep needed, the degree to which privacy is desired, and the extent to which the home situation is considered pleasant in the evenings distinguish best between the late group and the other two groups.

Indeed, examination of group means shows that the early and the on time groups claim to need more sleep ($\overline{X} = 2$ and $\overline{X} = 1.9$ respectively on the five-point Lickert scale where a score of 1 indicated total agreement) than the late group ($\overline{X} = 3$). The early group and the on time group need more privacy ($\overline{X} = 2.7$, $\overline{X} = 2.3$) than the

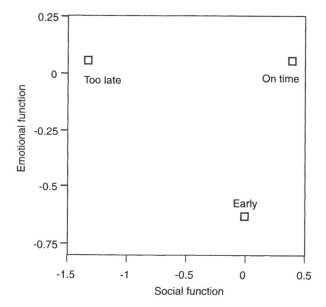

FIG. 8.1   Plot of 3 group centriods on 2 discriminant functions derived from 7 items concerning the meaning of sleep behaviour.

TABLE 8.1

Correlations between items and canonical discriminant functions
for sleeping behaviour

Item		Function 1	Function 2
1.	I do (or do not) need the sleep	−.53*	.26
2.	I want (or don't want) privacy	.47*	.23
3.	It is (or is not) cosy	.45*	−.11
4.	Being busy *vs.* having nothing to do	.30*	.09
5.	Does (not) help to deal with feeling rotten	−.19*	.05
6.	Does (not) help to deal with anger	−.12	.63*
7.	It is (or is not) healthy	.23	.51*
8.	Does (not) help to deal with frustration	.03	.23*
9.	Does (not) help to deal with being nervous	.02	.20*
10.	Parental demand *vs.* own decision	.07	.09*
	Canonical R	.57	.18
	Eigenvalue	.487	.032
	Wilk's lambda	.65	.97

late group ($\bar{X} = 3.3$). The late group gives staying up in the evenings higher scores on the cosiness continuum (late $\bar{X} = 3.8$, on time $\bar{X} = 4.5$, early $\bar{X} = 4.4$). The second discriminant function was not significant, so interpretation of group means is less secure. The early group scored somewhat higher on going to bed as a way of dealing with anger and on going to bed as a healthy, desirable behaviour. In discriminant analysis, the variables that best describe group differences are selected. The selection rule used here allowed only the variables that significantly decrease Wilks's lambda to be entered into the equation. Items 5, 9, and 10 did not meet this criterion and were not entered into the equation. For sleeping habits, 78.10% of the cases were correctly classified into one of the three groups using seven items representing the meaning of behaviour.

Eating habits at lunch time

The second analysis predicted membership in three groups representing eating habits at lunchtime. The classification procedure included five items describing the meaning of the behaviours. Of the original sample of 416 cases, 25 were excluded due to missing data and 391 cases were included in the analysis. Actual group membership was: lunch skippers ($n = 23$, 6%), healthy eaters (sandwiches, fruit, vegetables, $n = 262$, 67%), and junk food, snack foods, and sweets eaters ($n = 108$, 27%). Missing values were not randomly distributed over the three groups, with a greater proportion of missing data in the lunch skippers group. Prediction was not improved or impaired more than 2% by including user missing values as valid scores or by using estimated mean values. Cases with missing values were therefore excluded.

Two discriminant functions were derived, with a combined χ^2 (10) = 126.86, $p < .001$. After removal of the first function, there was still highly significant discriminating power, χ^2 (4) = 19. 69, $p < .001$. The two discriminant functions accounted for 86% and 14% of the between-group variability, respectively. As shown in Fig. 8.2, the first discriminant function (interpreted as the independence function) separates the junk food group from the healthy eaters, with the lunch skippers falling between the two, while the second function (interpreted as the feast or famine function) separates the lunch skippers from the other two groups.

The loading matrix of correlations between predictor variables and discriminant functions is shown in Table 8.2. Eating habits as representing the continuum between parental demand and making one's own decisions, and eating habits as a way of dealing with feeling rotten distinguish best the junk food group from the healthy eaters. Satisfying (or having no) appetite and worries about one's figure separate the lunch skippers from the other two groups.

The healthy eaters give the field of tension between parental control and personal choice less import than the other two groups (healthy eaters $\bar{X} = 3.63$, junk food group $\bar{X} = 2.34$, lunch skippers $\bar{X} = 2.96$). The junk food group scores higher on perceiving eating as a way to deal with feeling rotten (junk food group $\bar{X} = 4.11$, healthy eaters $\bar{X} = 4.56$, lunch skippers $\bar{X} = 4.48$). In the second discriminant function, the lunch skippers associate eating with satisfying hunger less than the other two groups and have less appetite (lunch skippers $\bar{X} = 2.87$,

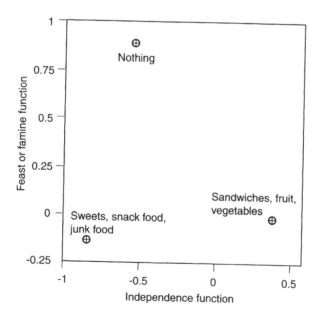

FIG. 8.2   Plot of 3 group centriods on 2 discriminant functions derived from 5 items concerning the meaning of eating behaviour at lunch.

TABLE 8.2

Correlations between items and canonical discriminant functions
for eating habits at lunch

Item	Function 1	Function 2
1. Parental demand *vs.* own decision	.78*	.23
2. Does (not) help to deal with feeling rotten	.35*	.27
3. Does (not) help to deal with anger	.30*	.22
4. Satisfy appetite *vs.* no desire for food	−.23	.91*
5. It is good (or bad) for my figure	.39	.47*
6. Does (not) help to deal with being nervous	.22	.24*
7. Does (not) help to deal with frustration	.22	.23*
8. It is (not) what everyone else does	−.12	.22*
Canonical R	.49	.22
Eigenvalue	.32	.052
Wilk's lambda	.72	.95

healthy eaters $\bar{X}$ = 1.80, junk food group $\bar{X}$ = 1.97). The lunch skippers claim that worries about their figure play little or no role in their lunch skipping behaviour, while the junk food group and the healthy eaters score higher on worries about their physique (lunch skippers $\bar{X}$ = 4.17, junk food group $\bar{X}$ = 3.43, healthy eaters $\bar{X}$ = 4.09). Items 3, 6, and 7 did not significantly decrease Wilks's lambda and were not entered into the equation. For eating behaviour at lunch, 74.30% of the cases could be classified correctly using five items representing the meaning of the behaviour.

Eating habits after school

The third discriminant analysis classified the subjects into three groups characterising eating habits after school. From the original sample of 416 subjects, 371 subjects were included in the analysis and 45 cases were excluded due to missing data. Actual group membership was: no food after school (n = 20, 5.33%), healthy eaters (sandwiches, fruit, vegetables, n = 101, 27.33%), and junk food and sweets eaters (n = 250, 67.33%). Missing values were not randomly distributed over the three groups, with a greater proportion of missing data in the abstainers group. Prediction was not improved or impaired more than 2% by including user-missing values or by using estimated mean values. Cases with missing values were therefore excluded.

Two discriminant functions were calculated, with a combined χ^2 (8) = 106.89, p < .001. After removal of the first function, discriminating power was still significant, χ^2 (3) = 47.96, p < .001. The two functions accounted for 55.5% and 44.5% of the between-group variability. As shown in Fig. 8.3, the first function (interpreted as the hunger function) separates the healthy eaters from the abstainers maximally, with the junk food group falling in between. The second function

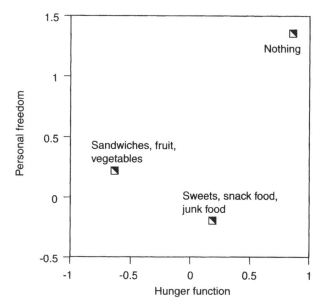

FIG. 8.3   Plot of 3 group centriods on 2 discriminant functions derived from 4 items concerning the meaning of eating behaviour after school.

(interpreted as the personal freedom function) separates the junk food group from the abstainers, with the healthy eaters in between.

The loading matrix as seen in Table 8.3 suggests that scores on the continuum between no appetite and a satisfaction of appetite distinguishes the abstainers from the healthy eaters. The continuum between parental demand and personal freedom, along with worries about the figure, distinguish the abstainers from the junk food group.

TABLE 8.3

Correlations between items and canonical discriminant functions for eating habits after school

Item		Function 1	Function 2
1.	Satisfy appetite *vs.* no desire for food	.83*	.56
2.	Does (not) help to deal with frustration	−.06*	.01
3.	Does (not) help to deal with anger	−.05*	.02
4.	Does (not) help to deal with being nervous	−.05*	−.02
5.	Parental demand *vs.* own decision	−.37	.85*
6.	It is good (or bad) for my figure	−.22	.38*
7.	Does (not) help to deal with feeling rotten	−.02	.08*
	Canonical R	.39	.35
	Eigenvalue	.176	.141
	Wilk's lambda	.75	.88

Group means reveal that hunger is less important for the abstainers ($\overline{X} = 3.3$) than for the healthy eaters ($\overline{X} = 1.5$), and plays a moderate role for the junk food group ($\overline{X} = 1.93$). The continuum between parental demand and personal freedom figures highly for the abstainers ($\overline{X} = 4.25$: on the low end of the scale is parental demands, on the high end of the scale is personal freedom, a score of 3 is neutral). The junk food group reports indifference on this continuum ($\overline{X} = 2.77$), while the healthy eaters tend towards making up their own minds ($\overline{X} = 3.67$). The junk food group scores higher on worries about one's figure than the other two groups (junk food group $\overline{X} = 3.6$, abstainers $\overline{X} = 4.2$, healthy eaters $\overline{X} = 4.05$). Items 3, 4, and 7 did not significantly decrease Wilks's lambda and were not entered into the equation. For eating behaviour at lunch, 69.27% of the cases could be classified correctly using four items representing the meaning of the behaviour.

DISCUSSION

For each of the three domains studied, between 69% and 78% of the behaviours could be predicted using items representing the meaning of that behaviour. These results are very encouraging, especially because predictive power has been achieved using only one construct.

For those who went to bed early and on time, the behaviour means getting enough sleep, but also represents privacy. For those who stay up too late, the payoff is a cosy atmosphere. In approaching the target group to improve sleeping habits (one out of five go to bed too late), emphasis might be placed on finding cosiness and companionship at another time of day and in other situations, on the need for sleep, and on the benefits of privacy and spending time alone.

At lunchtime, one-third of the group is engaging in less healthy behaviour. Eating junk food or skipping lunch represents asserting ones' own will, and the junk food group uses food as consolation. The abstainers are just not hungry, and do not report worrying about their figure. The junk food group does worry about their physique, as do the healthy eaters, but for the healthy eaters consuming healthy foods represents a way of taking care of their bodies. After school, more than two-thirds of the sample is eating junk food. Again, the abstainers are not hungry (only three subjects abstain both at lunch and after school, the groups are otherwise comprised of different subjects). The healthy eaters are ravenous, but the junk food eaters don't report hunger as a main motivation, and while they are eating unhealthy food, they are worrying about their figures. The abstainers report that eating nothing represents asserting their own will above that of their parents. Of course the connection between eating healthy foods and a pleasing body image deserves much attention in health education. Also, health education materials might redefine healthy dietary choices as self-assertive choices, and emphasise that poor eating habits do not, in the end, punish the parents.

One limitation of this study is that adolescence is treated as one stage in the analysis. However, differences in health habits between early and late adolescents have been found (see Chapter 7). Relevant for this study is that late adolescents (15 years and up) tend to get less sleep and make less healthy choices in diet (Cohen et al., 1990). Developmental tasks also differ for the two groups. Early adolescents must deal with puberty, changing sex roles, and the development of more autonomous relationships with parents and more mature relationships with peers. Late adolescents must prepare for adult work roles, evolve values to guide their behaviour, integrate their sexuality into their relationships, and achieve a sense of identity. It is thus feasible that salient meanings of these behaviours might also differ systematically for the two age groups. To examine this hypothesis, analyses must be carried out for early and late adolescents separately. The sample size did not permit separate analyses without violating the assumptions of discriminant analysis. Replication with a larger sample may offer some interesting insights.

Clear sex differences were found in eating behaviour after school (more girls eat junk food) and sleeping behaviour (more boys go to bed too late). Different meanings may be salient to the behaviour of the different sexes. To examine this hypothesis, analyses must be carried out for boys and girls separately. Once again, the sample size did not permit separate analyses, and replication with a larger sample is recommended. The possibility of an interaction between age and sex, in which four distinct groups would emerge, also deserves exploration. However, should determinants be different, and should these differences generate separate educational materials, implementation in a regular school system would present a number of practical problems.

It is unlikely that all salient meanings of behaviour were covered by the questionnaire. Further qualitative research into the different meanings of behaviour could enhance the predictive power, especially for eating habits after school. Finally, the research needs to be extended into other domains of health and risk behaviour, and to other ethic and cultural groups.

The results suggest that the perceived incentives construct of the model of Personal Investment may best be differentiated into intrinsic and extrinsic incentives, with the intrinsic meanings of behaviour representing the more affective determinants of behaviour. It remains to be seen how much predictive power is retained by extrinsic incentives. The possibility that intrinsic incentives far outweigh extrinsic incentives is an interesting one, and would entail re-examination of many of the central constructs in health behaviour research, such as the perceived barriers and perceived climate constructs.

These results were very exciting. They showed that personal, salient, and intrinsic meanings of behaviour could indeed be used successfully to predict that behaviour. Meanings exhibited good predictive power for eating and sleeping behaviours of adolescents. I could now assume that health and risk behaviours really do become imbued with affective meanings that are not connected to health-related knowledge or values. I could assume that these meanings indeed are determinants of the behaviours to which they become connected. Eating sweets might represent ways of comforting, rewarding, and punishing oneself. Skipping lunch takes on meanings of individuation, exercising personal will, assuming or rejecting personal responsibility, testing personal boundaries, and challenging authority. With this exploration of the predictive powers of salient meanings of behaviour, the fifth goal of the quantitative phase of the research had been accomplished. Theoretically, we could say that health-related behaviours were imbued with personal meanings, and that these meanings were in turn determinants of that behaviour. But could this predictive power be used in the field as a basis for effective health education and interventions? The next challenge was to see if this theory held up in practice.

PART FOUR

Applied research: Changing adolescent health-related behaviour

Effectiveness of an adolescent health education programme based on the Theory of the Meaning of Behaviour

Co-author: Rob J. Spruijt

INTRODUCTION

Three phases of research had now been completed, a theoretical one, a qualitative one, and a quantitative one. This final phase of the study is an applied one, where results of the first three stages are put to use and tested in the field. In this chapter, the process of development, implementation, and evaluation of a health education programme based on the research in the first three phases of the study is described.

What had we learned that could contribute to the development of relevant and effective health education for adolescents? The adolescent population exhibited a fairly broad knowledge base on health and health-related behaviour. However, this knowledge did not seem to translate well from the abstract to the concrete, and was often not seen as applicable to their own personal behaviour (Chapter 5). While girls and boys reported basically the same symptoms, the girls reported more symptoms and the boys reported better general health (Chapter 6). These gender differences were predominantly differences of degree rather than structural differences. This indicated that boys and girls might be able to profit from the same educational materials. The major areas of concern were also of similar content and structure between the boys and girls. While personal health was not directly experienced as a having a high priority, many top priorities were health-related. For instance, good personal appearance and high academic achievement were extremely important for both the boys and the girls (Chapter 6). They were also aware that eating junk food could have negative influences on personal appearance, and that getting too little sleep could have negative effects on academic achievement. However, this knowledge did not seem to affect behaviour (Chapter 7).

The focus group data (Chapter 5) suggested that adolescents tended to imbue everyday health-related behaviours with personal meanings that were not necessarily linked to health, and this had been substantiated in the survey (Chapter 8). Behaviours were imbued with meanings and came to represent not only certain behavioural objectives and outcomes, but also personal incentives that were completely intrinsic, having to do with feelings and fantasies. For instance, health-related behaviour could come to mean rebellion against authority, an expression of self-image, a way of dealing with anger or frustration, or a method of comforting, rewarding, or punishing oneself. These meanings were often disassociated from available knowledge of proximal behavioural outcomes, such as the knowledge that staying up late leads to fatigue the next day, and from knowledge of distal behavioural outcomes, such as the knowledge that eating quantities of sweets and junk food causes weight gain. In addition to the fact that meanings of behaviour were frequently unrelated to available knowledge of behavioural effects on health, they often took precedence over this knowledge as motivators of health-related behaviour. Perhaps because of this, salient meanings of behaviour had proven to be strong affect-based predictors of adolescent health-related behaviour (Chapter 8). Theoretically, this meant that behavioural changes might be accomplished indirectly by influencing corresponding salient meanings. The question remained, could this theory be used in practice? Could the predictive power of salient meanings of behaviour be of use prescriptively? The survey research (Chapter 8) had shown that there was a correlation between meanings of behaviour and actual behaviour. The challenge now was to see if that correlation indicated a causal relationship. Could meanings of behaviour be manipulated? And if so, would changes in meanings of a specific behaviour lead to changes in that behaviour? In order to answer these questions, the theory had to be tested in the field, embedded in health education materials. This chapter traces the design, implementation, and evaluation of a health education programme developed for the high-school classroom based on a theory of salient meanings of behaviour. This theory postulates that if we know the salient meanings that become attached to a particular behaviour by a specific target group, and we can change these meanings, the behaviour will follow suit.

Conceptually, healthy behaviours and risky behaviours are often considered to be related, and to share a single dimension where a particular risky behaviour represents one end of the scale, and a particular healthy behaviour the other. If more healthy food is eaten, it stands to reason and logic that less unhealthy food will be consumed. However, while these types of healthy and risky behaviours may be conceptually related, they often lack a simple linear empirical relationship (Chapter 8). We saw that risky behaviours tended to cluster and healthy behaviours could function as general buffers against risky ones, but an inverse relationship between conceptually juxtaposed health and risk behaviours was not always present. Change in one behaviour will therefore not automatically have repercussions for another, conceptually related behaviour, because it might not live on the other end of an imaginary scale. For these reasons, behavioural objectives for health education interventions must be clearly defined. While information on the down side of relevant unhealthy behaviours is also supplied to ensure a comprehensive and relevant education, the lesson materials created for this research are primarily designed to enhance targeted health behaviours. It is hypothesised that use of the lesson materials will influence salient meanings of targeted behaviours, which will in turn lead to behaviour change. We expect that behaviour change will be evidenced principally by an increase in healthy behaviours.

In order to test the theory in the field, three strategies were devised to approach behavioural change indirectly, through attempting to shift meanings of behaviour. These could be used in conjunction or separately, depending upon the behavioural objectives and the meanings themselves. The first strategy was to connect salient meanings with behavioural objectives. Socially acceptable or positively valued meanings of behaviour, such as independence and self-esteem, could be used to encourage healthy behaviours by showing how these behaviours are related to such salient meanings. Conversely, risky behaviours could perhaps be discouraged if it could be convincingly demonstrated that they were negatively related to salient meanings. The second approach was to transform accepted knowledge-related meanings into salient meanings and then to connect them with behavioural objectives. This involved increasing the value of meanings of behaviour that are known to be of little influence in the target group, such as healthiness, and then connecting these meanings with behavioural objectives. A third approach was to reduce the salience of meanings that were already connected with behaviour. In this case, meanings that obstructed behavioural objectives, such as the connection made by many teenage girls between skipping lunch at school and having a beautiful body, were discredited and their connection with behaviour was weakened.

METHODS AND MATERIALS

Construction of the lesson materials

To construct the lesson materials, the domains of everyday health-related behaviour relevant for the target group had to be determined, behavioural objectives had to be established, and salient meanings of the behaviours involved needed to be ascertained. Furthermore, guiding principles from the many available pedagogical and educational ideologies needed to be selected and implemented.

Determining relevant domains of health. From the focus group interviews (Chapter 5) and open questionnaire (Chapter 4) hypotheses had been generated concerning which health issues were important for Dutch adolescents, how they relate to health in general, what they know about everyday healthy and risky behaviours, and the determinants of health-related behaviours in this population. These hypotheses had then been refined and tested in the survey (Chapters 6, 7, and 8). Four domains in everyday health emerged from this research as areas in which the adolescents felt that there was room for improvement in their own behaviour, and where they reported the need for help in making appropriate changes through better, more relevant information. These domains were: nutrition, sleep and rest, physical symptoms such as headaches and coughs, and communication skills including talking about their problems.[1] One aspect of nutrition, beverage consumption and thirst, was chosen as the central topic for the lesson materials designed for this research.

A major criticism of many health education programmes is that they are often not systematic, sequenced, or comprehensive, and that they treat different (but related) issues at different times, thereby ignoring important relationships (Boekaerts, & Simons, 1993; Froman, & Owen, 1991). To avoid these limitations, all four of the domains receive attention in the lesson materials, their interrelations are described, and relevant relationships with other areas of health and well-being are touched upon. Figure 9.1 is an excerpt from the lesson materials showing how aspects of nutrition, rest, physical symptoms, and communication skills have been integrated and related. This and all subsequent excerpts from the lesson materials are translations from the original Dutch.

Establishing behavioural objectives. Establishing nutritionally sound behavioural objectives for daily liquid intake proved to be a complex undertaking. Textbooks on nutrition often disagreed upon such basic issues as calcium intake, sugar intake, the safe level of various additives, and suggested intake of litres per day (Clark, Parr, & Castelli, 1988; Elmadia & Muskat, 1992; Hamilton et al., 1991; Hendrikz, & de Moor, 1982; Katch, & McArdle, 1993; Nutricia, 1984; Pipes, & Trahms, 1993; Sizer, & Whitney, 1997). Advice was often not differentiated or tailored to the special needs of adolescents (Clark et al., 1988; Cobb, 1992; Pipes, & Trahms, 1993). Formal advice from the Ministry of Health was not always in accordance with the textbooks, and the Dutch, American, and Canadian advice differs on several issues (Hamilton et al., 1991; Voorlichting voor de Voeding, 1993; Voedingsraad, 1986). To circumvent these controversies and formulate state-of-the-art nutrition guidelines, a self-administered, open and closed question survey (Fowler, 1993) was developed using information from informal interviews with nutrition experts, textbooks, existing lesson material, and government publications. The survey was conducted with nutritionists, dieticians, general practitioners, and researchers in the area of human nutrition. While agreement on key issues was not forthcoming, the quality of the argumentation and the relative frequency of various

---

[1]Concerning this last domain, it is interesting to note that while research on the health influences of disclosure has only recently gained momentum and a broader acceptance in the scientific community (Pennebaker, 1990), the Dutch adolescents seem to intuitively accept the relevance of disclosure for their own health.

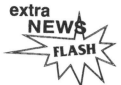

Be where you want to be when you want to be there!

If you don't want to miss important stuff, at school or after school, you've got to be able to count on your body to get you there. But this means that your body has got to be able to count on YOU!

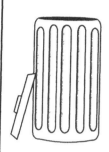
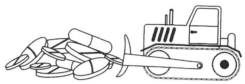

So listen to your body, it has a lot to say. If you feel symptoms of a cold or flu coming on, make sure that you get enough to drink, dress warmly if it is cold outside, and get enough rest! This gives you the best chance that the cold or flu won't take hold, and that your health won't mess up any of your plans! And if you really do get a fever and you have to miss something important, take care of yourself and don't expose everyone to your germs!

Ask your friends to take notes for you or take care of any important business for you, and stay home in bed. You need to be able to trust your body, and it is also important to be able to trust your friends to help you out in a tight spot! Just like it is a two way street between you and your friends, it is a two way street between you and your body. Taking care goes in both directions.

FIG. 9.1   Excerpt from the lesson materials integrating four areas of health behaviour.

opinions found in the completed questionnaires facilitated the construction of up-to-date lesson materials and ensured the setting of sound behavioural goals.

Determining salient meanings of behaviour and their relationships to that behaviour. In order to be predictive of behaviour, meanings must be salient to the population. The salient meanings of behaviours related to nutrition were established using data from the focus groups and the survey, and extrapolated to the specific beverage consumption behaviours studied here. Manipulations of meanings were presented as 'extra news flashes' in the materials. Three strategies were employed in the 'extra news flashes' to influence meanings, corresponding to the postulated relationships between meanings and behaviour. Figures 9.2–9.4 are English translations from the Dutch lesson material illustrating each of these three strategies. The strategies were often used simultaneously, as is evidenced in the examples. Figure 9.2 shows an extra news flash in which behavioural objectives (drinking more fruit juice) are attached to salient meanings (independence). In Fig. 9.3, accepted, knowledge-related meanings (healthiness, cause and effect) are attached

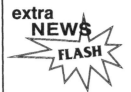

Can I make some of my own choices around here?

You share the responsibility for your health with your parents and your community. At home, your parents probably do the shopping and cooking most of the time. At school, you learn about healthy behaviours (like in this book), but you also see many unhealthy behaviours. Your choices are also influenced by whatever foods and drinks are easily available, and by what your friends eat and drink. And of course business and advertising do their very best to control your choices and your tastes!

Whoever is trying to influence you, the final responsibility for what you eat and drink is YOURS! You can take this responsibility by using this lesson material wisely, and by making smart and independent choices. Here are a few tips for getting your own health together by taking the responsibility you are ready for:

1. Tell your parents what you would like them to buy at the market—ask, for instance, for oranges for juice instead of soft drinks!

2. Help make the shopping lists.

3. Make your OWN choices in the cafeteria at school! Don't eat and drink anything just because other people do it or because you have seen it advertised on television!

4. Ask for your own food budget.

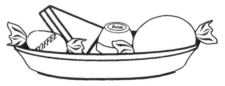

Can you think of other ways to get more control over what you eat and drink?

FIG. 9.2   Special news flash attaching behavioural objectives to salient meanings.

to behavioural objectives (drinking more milk and less chocolate milk) and we then attempt to make these meanings salient. In Fig. 9.4, an attempt is made to reduce the salience of certain meanings (choice of drinks represents the expression of personal taste) and weaken their relationship with behaviours (drinking popular drinks, especially soft drinks).

Selecting and implementing didactic principles. The vision of human learning upon which the lesson materials were based is an amalgamation of the ideas from Gagné (Gagné, & Briggs, 1979), Boekaerts and Simons (1993), and Broekman (Broekman et al., 1993). The lesson materials aim at teaching health skills through emphasising three aspects of those skills. These are (1) feeling (emotion), (2) thinking and knowing (cognition), and (3) taking action (behaviour). Feeling pertains to perception of physical sensations and interpreting these signals sensibly.

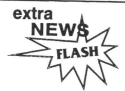

While you could say that grasping the relationships between causes and effects is our most important tool for understanding our world, we are notoriously lousy at it. Why?

1. When we feel something, we automatically look for the cause in events that took place directly before the feeling: a few minutes, or at most a few hours before. If you feel a headache coming on in the afternoon, you will blame the fact that you didn't eat or drink enough in the last few hours, didn't get enough sleep the night before, or maybe you just had an argument with someone. People hardly ever look for explanations for what they feel in something that they might have done a few weeks, months, or years ago. But what you did last week, last month and last year can have a lot of influence on your health today (check out the crossword puzzle, for instance, to understand the influence of the calcium in your diet now on your health later on).

2. Another reason that we are pretty lousy at understanding connections between causes and effects is because we tend to ignore things that we would rather not have to deal with for one reason or another. Sometimes we hide the consequences of our behaviour from others, and sometimes we even try to fool ourselves about them. For instance, you know that it is better for you not to drink that second carton of chocolate milk. But you don't pay any attention to that knowledge, and only after you drink it do you end up feeling guilty, sorry, or nauseous.

Did you know that understanding the relationships between what you do and how you feel can help you to change your habits and to feel healthier? Keep in mind that what you do today can have consequences for how you feel next week, next month, and even in a few years!

FIG. 9.3   Special news flash associating accepted meanings with behavioural objectives.

This entails being able to recognise various sensations such as hunger, thirst, and tiredness, and recognising one's own limits and when they have been reached. Thinking and knowing represent not only the knowledge component and awareness of cause and effect, but also applying knowledge to physical sensations. This includes being able to recognise when a symptom can be dealt with privately, when professional help is needed, and how to formulate relevant questions to get the knowledge needed. Taking action entails being able to undertake appropriate behaviours, to use knowledge to make independent choices, and to back up health-related choices with sound arguments. This includes being able to communicate clearly about personal health questions or problems, and knowing where and how to get any information and help that might be needed.

Research with cognitively active students such as the participants in this study (college preparatory high school) shows that these students function better in a

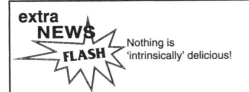

Nothing is 'intrinsically' delicious!

You *learn* to like things. Nothing is "intrinsically" delicious to everyone. Soft drinks, coffee, orange juice, milk: if you like them, you *learned* to like them. You learn to like things in several ways, and for several reasons:

1. You recognise it:
   If you see something often enough at home, on T.V., or at friends houses, you are more likely to recognise it and to try it out. If you try it often enough, you will probably learn to like it. This is one of the basic principles of T.V., radio, and other media advertising. What you think you 'naturally' like is determined, influenced, and changed by the fact that you learn to recognise food products by seeing them often enough.

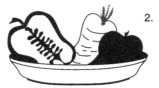

2. It is familiar:
   If a product is used regularly in the home, you not only learn to recognise it, you become *familiar* with it. If family members or friends like a certain food product, there is a big chance that you will also learn to like it.

3. It is easy to get:
   If a certain food or drink is easy to get at school or in the local store, you are more likely to buy it. Simple but true.

Now, have you chosen this product yourself, or was it easier to learn to like it than to resist it?

What now? *Think* before you choose and then make up your own mind. Eating and drinking can be a real adventure, or just something that is familiar, the usual stuff. But remember, there is no such thing as 'naturally delicious'. You *learn* to like things. That means you can change your own tastes by teaching yourself to like other things if *you* decide to. And THAT means that healthy food and drink *can* be one and the same as delicious food and drink! It is up to you!

FIG. 9.4   Special news flash reducing the salience of meanings and weakening their relationship with behaviours.

situation which affords them the freedom to take their own initiative, plan their own activities, and which stimulates them to use their own knowledge and capacities (Boekaerts, & Simons, 1993). Therefore, the different sections in the lesson materials do not have a prescribed order and can be worked through independently in the order chosen by each student according to his or her interests or preferences. A variety of didactic forms are used in the lesson materials to promote learning health skills (Boekaerts, & Simons, 1993). The games, exercises, experiments and puzzles are prefaced by a short 'News Flash' in which a few of the most relevant facts on the topic are given along with instructions. In each section, the puzzles and games are given *before* the material is discussed in detail. Questions in the puzzles and games challenge the students to induce answers from their own existing knowledge before they receive the bulk of the instruction. The answers, in which the bulk of the instruction is found, *follow* the exercises.

Because positive messages are more likely to motivate behaviour change than negative mandates and fear messages (Eagly, & Chaiken, 1993; Petty, & Cacioppo, 1986), the lesson materials predominantly employ positive messages on the good effects of healthy behaviour. Lastly, extra attention was paid to graphics and design. The kind of first impression that lesson materials make is determined by their appearance. A good first impression contributes to the motivation to use the materials (Boekaerts, & Simons, 1993) . We strove to create an attractive package that was reminiscent neither of regular school materials nor of commercial pamphlets.

Participants

Twelve classes from three different college preparatory high schools in The Netherlands took part in this study, a total of 325 students (168 girls and 157 boys). The ages of the participants ranged from 11 to 15 years, with a mean age of 13.26 years. Several biology and social science teachers from college preparatory secondary schools in North Holland were formally invited to participate in the research. Four teachers who gained permission from the heads of their schools and felt that the subject matter fit into their curriculum participated.

Design

A Solomon four-group design was chosen for this study (Kidder, & Judd, 1986; Tones, & Tilford, 1994). To ascertain if any behavioural changes are attributable to manipulations of meanings of behaviour rather than to other aspects of the lesson materials, two versions of the lesson materials were prepared. One version of the materials included eight special sections emphasising the meanings of behaviours as illustrated above (treatment M/meanings). In the second version of the materials, the special sections on meanings were deleted and replaced with computer art (treatment NM/no meanings). In all other aspects, the second version was identical to the first. Six classes used the materials with the special sections on meanings, six used the materials without the special sections. In the Solomon four-group design, half of each treatment group is pre-tested on relevant measures, and half is not. This yields four groups (Table 9.1). All four groups are post-tested.

Procedure

Four lessons on nutrition were given over a period of two weeks using the lesson materials on beverage consumption and thirst. These lessons were given by biology or social studies teachers as part of the regular curriculum. To avoid spurious effects

TABLE 9.1

The Solomon four-group design

Group 1	Pretest	treatment M/meanings	Post-test
Group 2	No pretest	treatment M/meanings	Post-test
Group 3	Pretest	treatment NM/no meanings	Post-test
Group 4	No pretest	treatment NM/no meanings	Post-test

due to possible differences in teaching style, each of the four participating teachers gave classes using both sets of materials, and was instructed to avoid using material or ideas from the special sections in the treatment NM classes.

On the first day of the study, half of each class was pre-tested on extant knowledge about nutrition, beverage consumption and the meanings of those behaviours, while the other half filled in a questionnaire of comparable length from an entirely unrelated study. Each participating student was given a 'beverage consumption diary' and instructions on using the diary to keep track of the type and amount of daily liquid consumption for the first week of the study. The entire sample completed a 33-question post-test during class within one week after the last lesson on beverage consumption and thirst. The pre-tests and the post-tests were identical, thus all measures were taken at pre-test and repeated at post-test, except for demographic data concerning age, school, cultural background and gender which was gathered at post-test only. After completion of the post-tests, focus group interviews were conducted with six students from each class who volunteered to participate, and informal interviews were done with the teachers to evaluate their experiences with the materials.

Variables

Seven *dependent variables* were included in this study: knowledge about nutrition, the amount of milk, fruit juice, chocolate milk, sugared soft drinks, coffee consumed, and a total score for healthy behaviour. Knowledge about nutrition was measured by summing the number of correctly answered questions out of 10 multiple choice questions on nutrition. A five-point Likert-type scale was used to assess consumption of the five drinks (1 = never drink it, 2 = a few glasses (or cups) a month, 3 = 1–3 glasses a week, 4 = 4–7 glasses a week, and 5 = more than seven glasses a week). To calculate the total score for healthy behaviour, the Likert scales for the three less healthy drinks (chocolate milk, soft drinks, and coffee) were reversed (so that 5 = never drink it, 4 = a few glasses a month, and so forth), and the scores for all five drinks were summed. In this way, a high total score indicated high consumption of the healthy drinks *and* low consumption of the less healthy drinks.

The *mediating variables* in this study are the meanings of each behaviour, which are hypothesised to influence that behaviour. Eleven possible salient meanings for all the dependent variables were generated using material from the focus group interviews. These meanings included such items as 'I drink [juice, soft drinks, etc.] because it helps me deal with my anger', 'I drink [juice, soft drinks, etc.] because my parents don't [or do] want me to', or 'I drink [juice, soft drinks, etc.] because it is healthy'. Meanings were scored for consuming as well as abstaining from consumption. Because the study of meanings of behaviour is still being developed, no a priori choices were made as to which meaning would be salient for which drink. All eleven meanings were scored on a five-point Likert-type scale for each of the behaviours (1= totally agree to 5 = totally disagree). The lower the score, the more salient the meaning.

It was hypothesised that the meanings of behaviour would in turn be manipulated or influenced by the *treatment conditions*: treatment M being the lesson materials *with* special sections on the meanings of behaviour, and treatment NM being the lesson materials *without* the special sections on the meanings of behaviour. Because gender differences on health-related behaviours are the rule rather than the exception, gender will be included in all the analyses as a *classification factor,* yielding a $2 \times 2 \times 2$ factorial design (pre-test/no pre-test, boy/girl, treatment NM/treatment M).

Statistical analyses

The beverage consumption diaries served as descriptive material to illustrate the overall beverage consumption of the population.

Initial $2 \times 2 \times 2$ ANOVAs showed significant interactions between pre-test and treatment on several of the behaviours, indicating that pre-test sensitisation had occurred. Examination of cell means indicated that the subjects who were pre-tested reacted less favourably to the treatment than those who were not. These findings were corroborated in the focus group interviews, in which the pre-test was repeatedly evaluated as negative, demotivating, and lacking in any evident context. The occurrence of pre-test sensitisation indicates that treatment effects cannot be isolated from pre-test effects in the subjects who were pre-tested. Undergoing the pre-test influenced the effects of the treatment for these subjects. As the main concern of this research was the effects of the lesson materials themselves, further analyses are carried out using only the scores from the treatment NM and treatment M groups who did *not* undergo a pre-test (169 subjects: 88 girls and 81 boys). Thus, all further analyses reported here (except the descriptive statistics for the beverage consumption diaries) involve *post-test* scores only.

While ANOVAs imply two-tailed testing, one-tailed testing was called for to test the hypotheses concerning the effects of the treatment. Because only two independent treatment levels were compared, the relationship $F = t^2$ could be used to compute a t-value which will be used for one-sided testing.

To establish if the different treatments had differential effects on learning, an ANOVA was conducted with knowledge about nutrition as the dependent variable. Correlations between the five behaviours were then examined. To investigate possible treatment effects, gender differences, and interaction effects, ANOVAs were used with the total score for healthy beverage consumption and each of the five beverage consumption behaviours as dependent variables. If effects of the treatment on behaviours were detected in these ANOVAs, it had to be demonstrated that these effects were due to treatment-induced differences in meanings of behaviour. Therefore, ANCOVAs were performed, with the behaviours as dependent variables and the scores for their meanings as covariates. If the changes in behaviours were indeed due to changes in their respective meanings, there should be no independent effect of the treatment (and of gender) on behaviour.[2] Figure 9.5 demonstrates the procedure.

With the ANOVAs, differences between the treatment groups in behaviour are demonstrated without the mediating effect of the meanings (solid line). In the ANCOVAs, all differences demonstrated with the ANOVAs should be attributed to the differences in meanings. Hence, the covariates should show significant effects on the behaviour (second dotted line), while no (independent) effects of the treatment on the behaviours should remain (solid line). The effects of the treatment on the meanings (first dotted line) are not demonstrated separately, but are implied if the meanings subsume an independent treatment effect on the behaviours (solid line).

RESULTS

The diaries

The seven-day beverage consumption diary was completed by 285 subjects (149 girls and 136 boys). The 40 students who did not complete the beverage consumption diaries were spread equally over the participating classes and ages by year. Reasons given for not turning in a completed diary were absence or loss. From the students who did complete the diaries, the girls reported drinking less (an average of 1.3 litres a day) than the boys (1.6 litres a day; Behrends–Fisher

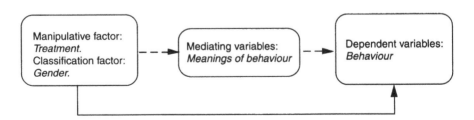

FIG. 9.5   Testing the influence of factors and mediating variables using ANOVA and ANCOVA.

---

[2]For a discussion of the robustness of ANOVA and ANCOVA when using Likert-type scales, see van der Kamp et al. (1992).

$t = -4.33$; df = 242.17; $P < .00$). The diaries were mentioned frequently in the focus groups. The subjects found it very revealing to keep track of what they drank, and reported temporary changes in their behaviour as a result:

> It is incredibly frustrating to see how much sweet junk I really drink. I really started being more careful after I saw that on paper.

> I really drank more, and more milk and water and fewer soft drinks, because I had to write it down.

Figure 9.6 shows the mean reported consumption of each of the drinks in the diary for girls and boys in litres per day.

ANOVAs and ANCOVAs

There were no univariate or multivariate outliers, and results of evaluation of the assumptions of normality, linearity, homogeneity of regression and reliability of covariates were satisfactory. No difference in knowledge about nutrition was found between the two treatment groups ($F = .015$; df = 1, 165, $p = .9$). The girls scored higher on knowledge than the boys (girls = 5.74, boys 5.14; $F = 5.71$; df = 1, 165; $p = .02$). There was no interaction effect between treatment and gender ($F = .03$; df = 1, 165; $p = .87$).

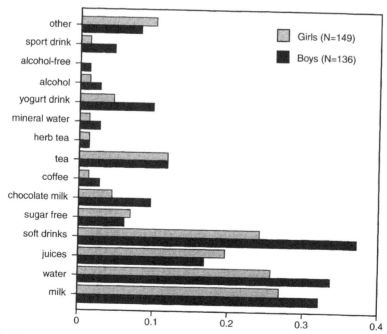

FIG. 9.6   Beverage consumption of girls and boys in litres per day.

No significant correlations were found between the five beverage consumption behaviours (drinking fruit juice, milk, soft drinks, chocolate milk, and coffee). The treatment M group with the meanings included in the material scored higher on overall healthy beverage consumption (treatment NM = 14.45, treatment M = 15.52). The ANOVA for total healthy beverage consumption scores showed a significant treatment effect ($F = 6.19$; df = 1, 153; $p < .01$, one-tailed). No significant effects of gender or the interaction between gender and treatment were found. The results of the ANOVAs on the post-test scores of the five separate drinks appear in Table 9.2.

After the four lessons using the lesson material described here, the treatment M group with the sections on the meanings of behaviour included in their materials reported drinking more juice (treatment NM = 3.29, treatment M = 3.71) and more milk (treatment NM = 3.46, treatment M = 4.07) than the treatment NM group without the special sections. The treatment M group also reported drinking less chocolate milk (treatment NM = 4.11, treatment M = 3.76). No treatment effects were found for soft drinks or coffee. Significant gender differences were found for fruit juice and soft drinks. The girls in both treatment groups drink more fruit juice than the boys in both groups. The boys drink more soft drinks.

To determine whether the detected treatment effects could be attributed to shifts in the meaning of behaviour, ANCOVAs were carried out for the three behaviours in which treatment effects were found. The sample size dictates that no more than five covariates be included in each analysis (Stevens, 1992). Meanings that showed significant (partial) correlation with the behaviour in question were considered for

TABLE 9.2

ANOVAs for the effect of treatment and gender on drinking behaviours

Behaviour	Effect	df	F
Drinking fruit juice	Treatment	1,162	4.00[c]
	Gender	1,162	6.10[a]
	Interaction	1,162	.90
Drinking milk	Treatment	1,164	4.40[c]
	Gender	1,164	.57
	Interaction	1,164	.04
Drinking and soft drinks	Treatment	1,164	.07
	Gender	1,164	5.11[a]
	Interaction	1,164	.49
Drinking chocolate milk	Treatment	1,163	3.74[b]
	Gender	1,163	.54
	Interaction	1,163	2.54
Drinking chocolate	Treatment	1,158	.02
	Gender	1,158	2.05
	Interaction	1,158	.98

[a] Significant at $p < .05$, two-tailed test.
[b] Significant at $p < .05$, one-tailed test.
[c] Significant at $p < .025$, one-tailed test.

the analyses. Interestingly, the knowledge about nutrition scores showed no correlation with the behaviours, and were therefore omitted from further analyses. The results of the ANCOVAs are shown in Table 9.3.

As hypothesised, the main effects of the treatment on drinking fruit juice, milk, and chocolate milk are due to treatment-induced differences in meanings. The meanings of behaviour also explain gender differences in drinking fruit juice. In Table 9.4, the post-test mean scores are given for the meanings which showed significant effects in the ANCOVAs.

Healthiness and availability have become more salient for the treatment M groups for both healthy behaviours. For drinking fruit juice, the expression of

TABLE 9.3

ANCOVAs for the effect of the manipulation of meanings of behaviours

Behaviour	Effect	df	F
Drinking fruit juice	Covariates	5,162	10.08**
	Personal taste	1,162	15.41**
	Availability	1,162	8.67**
	Healthy	1,162	5.34*
	Spoil oneself	1,162	.26
	Body image	1,162	.54
	Main effects	2,162	2.06
	Treatment	1,162	2.62
	Gender	1,162	1.34
	Interactions	1,162	2.50
Drinking milk	Covariates	5,152	15.03**
	Personal taste	1,152	.03
	Body image	1,152	1.55
	Healthy	1,152	13.64**
	Availability	1,152	5.62*
	Beautiful teeth	1,152	2.5
	Main effects	2,152	1.27
	Treatment	1,152	1.06
	Gender	1,152	1.62
	Interactions	1,152	.15
Drinking chocolate milk	Covariates	5,152	14.47**
	Gives energy	1,152	19.71**
	Personal taste	1,152	14.84**
	Body image	1,152	16.02**
	Rebellion	1,152	.87
	Spoil myself	1,152	7.74**
	Main effects	2,152	.40
	Treatment	1,152	.08
	Gender	1,152	.71
	Interactions	1,152	.34

*Significant at $p < .025$.
**Significant at $p < .01$.

TABLE 9.4

Mean scores on the meanings that explain main effects of treatment and gender*

Variable	$\bar{X}$ treatment = NM	$\bar{X}$ treatment = M
Main effect treatment:		
Fruit juice		
Personal taste	2.01	1.59
Availability	2.54	2.35
Healthy	2.61	2.29
Milk		
Availability	3.14	2.89
Healthy	2.35	2.05
Chocolate milk		
Body sensations	3.67	3.80
Personal taste	2.26	1.94
Body image	4.04	3.84
Spoil myself	3.42	3.25
	$\bar{X}$ girls	$\bar{X}$ boys
Main effect gender:		
Fruit juice		
Personal taste	1.63	1.97
Availability	2.37	2.53
Healthy	2.30	2.62

*The lower the score, the more salient the meaning.

personal taste has also become more salient for the treatment M group. For drinking chocolate milk, a different set of meanings show significant effects, with the exception of personal taste. The item on body sensations refers to experiencing an energy boost as a reason to drink chocolate milk and experiencing an unpleasant, over-full sensation as a reason to avoid it. The higher score on the item in the treatment M group indicates that drinking chocolate milk was experienced as unpleasant more often by this group. Body image and personal taste have become salient reasons to abstain from drinking chocolate milk for the treatment M group. Perhaps because they now drink it less often, drinking chocolate milk has become a way of spoiling oneself for this group. Where gender differences in drinking fruit juice are concerned, healthiness, availability, and the expression of personal taste are generally more salient for the girls than for the boys.

DISCUSSION

At the end of a two-week trial, the treatment group exposed to lesson materials *with* special sections on the meanings of behaviour reported drinking more fruit juice, more milk, and less chocolate milk than the group exposed to lesson materials without these special sections. Differences were found between the two treatment groups in meanings of behaviour, but not in knowledge about nutrition. This confirms previous findings demonstrating that knowledge is not a major determinant of health-related behaviour (Becker et al., 1972; Glanz et al., 1990).The treatment effects were shown to be entirely due to the manipulations of the meanings of behaviour.

Three strategies for influencing salient meanings were implemented in the treatment: (1) attaching adolescents' salient meanings to targeted behaviour, (2) attaching non-salient accepted meanings to targeted behaviour and enhancing their salience, and (3) reducing the salience of obstructive meanings connected to targeted behaviours. There is evidence that all three strategies contributed to the effectiveness of the lesson materials. Using the first strategy, drinking fruit juice was associated with independence, so that fruit juice consumption came to mean an expression of personal taste and independence. From the focus groups, independence from parents had indeed emerged as one of the most salient meanings of both healthy and risky behaviours. Another example of the first strategy was the effective association of a desirable body image with decreased consumption of chocolate milk. The second strategy was used to enhance the salience of meanings related to healthiness and associate them with both milk and juice consumption. Healthiness was shown to be one of the least important concerns for this population (Chapter 6). The results show that both milk and juice consumption had come to represent healthy behaviour, and that this meaning had become salient enough to affect both milk and juice consumption positively. Strategy two was also used to influence the salience of availability and associate it with healthy behaviours. In the lesson materials including the sections on the meanings of behaviour, the subjects were encouraged to help with the shopping and share the responsibility for making healthy drinks available at home. In this way, the salience of availability was expanded and brought into the sphere of personal control and expression. Consequently, meanings associated with availability contributed to increased consumption of both milk and juice. An example of the use of the third strategy was the attempt made to play down the importance of personal taste in chocolate milk consumption. Not only was personal taste disassociated from chocolate milk consumption, it also became associated with abstaining from consumption of chocolate milk.

Consumption of chocolate milk was reduced, but the lesson materials affected neither soft drink nor coffee consumption. While the data from the beverage consumption diaries show that coffee consumption in this group is negligible, soft drinks remain popular. The treatment was, in general, more effective in enhancing healthy behaviours than in reducing unhealthy ones. This and the fact that no inter-relationships were found between the five beverage consumption behaviours studied here lends credence to the thesis that conceptually related healthy and risky behaviours do not always live on one continuum (Chapter 7). Changes in one behaviour cannot be expected to have repercussions for other, conceptually related behaviours. This means that the behavioural objectives for health education interventions must be set very specifically. Also, if conceptually related behaviours show no empirical relationship, a re-examination of our understanding of these behaviours may be in order.

The salience of meanings associated with personal taste, availability, and healthiness also accounted for the gender differences found in the consumption of fruit juice, independent of the treatment. This suggests that the meanings of some behaviours may differ for boys and girls. Gender difference in meanings of behaviour invites further study.

Taking a pre-test in this situation, without a context and without prior preparation, was not only experienced as negative by the subjects at the time of testing, but interfered with the effectiveness of the lesson materials for the duration of the study. This finding stresses the importance of research designs which allow for the detection of pre-test effects. It may also serve as a reminder for educators. Tests are effective treatments in and of themselves, and pre-testing students in order to obtain baseline measurements could, in some cases, affect subsequent performance.

The study was relatively short and no follow-up study was conducted to trace the persistence of the treatment effect. Therefore, this must be regarded as a pilot study. Its brief character mandates extreme caution in drawing any conclusions. Effective interventions within high-school populations require 'brush-ups' and 'booster sessions' at regular intervals to retain effects (Perry, & Kelder, 1992). The conditions most conducive to the persistence of behavioural effects achieved with this kind of lesson materials require further research.

Notwithstanding the brief character of the intervention, lesson materials based upon the meaning of behaviour contributed to an increase in healthy behaviour. Behavioural change was accomplished indirectly, by including messages designed to influence the meanings of the target behaviours. Our results conform to many earlier studies in that we once again find that the dissemination of knowledge is not enough to obtain behavioural change. However, let it not go unsaid that, in our opinion, it remains our responsibility as health educators to include up-to-date and relevant information as part and parcel of our interventions.

In this book, the trajectory of the development of theory on salient meanings of behaviour was traced through four phases of research. Its development was followed from hunch to idea to hypothesis to application. In this final, applied phase of the research, it was found that relevant and effective adolescent health education materials could be created using messages designed to influence the meanings of behaviour. Meanings of behaviour have thus been shown to be determinants of health-related behaviour in adolescence. With this, a journey through the empirical cycle was completed.

Concluding remarks

It is possible that the theory developed here is generalisable to other domains of behaviour than the ones studied here, both inside and outside the realm of health. Generalisability over time is an issue on several levels. As new health-related research findings are made available, different behaviours may become important for health and health education. Different sets of risky and healthy behaviours also emerge as new products, new fads, and new trends in behaviour appear. Salient meanings for extant behaviours may also change because adolescent concerns are subject to modification as cultural and historical contexts evolve. To use this theory effectively, periodic updates of interventions will most likely be required; both to accommodate the changing compendium of behaviours that are considered healthy or risky, and to accommodate changes in salient meanings. Study of gender, developmental and cultural differences in health behaviours and their respective meanings would contribute to the understanding of adolescent health-related behaviour and could improve the effectiveness of meaning-based interventions. Finally, this research was conducted exclusively for and with adolescents and premised on the need for less rationally based models of adolescent behaviour. The possibility that the meanings of behaviour may also predict adult health-related behaviour remains to be studied.

In this book, a specific methodology for the development of relevant and effective lesson materials for adolescents is unfolded and elucidated. Each of the four phases aided in the development of the theoretical framework based on the meanings with which adolescents tend to imbue health-related behaviour. The theory of salient meanings of behaviour developed in these pages might help us to gain insight into behaviour, to predict it, and to create effective health education interventions that bring about behavioural change. I hope this theory will offer a useful addition to the body of theory on determinants of adolescent health-related behaviour.

References

Abraham, C., Sheeran, P., Spears, R., & Abrams, D. (1992). Health beliefs and promotion of HIV-preventive intentions among teenagers: A Scottish perspective. *Health Psychology, 11,* 363–370.

Agresti, A. (1990). *Categorical data analysis.* New York: John Wiley & Sons.

Ajzen, I. (1985). From intentions to actions: A theory of planned behavior. In J. Kuhl & J. Beckman (Eds.), *Action control: From cognition to behavior* (pp. 11–39). New York: Springer-Verlag.

Ajzen, I. (1994). Lecture at the University of Amsterdam, The Netherlands.

Ajzen, I., & Fishbein, M. (1977). Attitude-behavior relations: A theoretical analysis and review of empirical research. *Psychological Bulletin, 84,* 888–918.

Ajzen, I., & Fishbein, M. (1980). *Understanding attitudes and predicting social behavior.* Englewood Cliffs, NJ: Prentice-Hall.

Ajzen, I., & Madden, J.T. (1986). Prediction of goal-directed behavior: Attitudes, intentions, and perceived behavior control. *Journal of Experimental Social Psychology, 22,* 453–474.

Alexander, C.S. (1989). Gender differences in adolescent health concerns and self assessed health. *Journal of Early Adolescence, 9,* 467–479.

Arbuckle, J.L. (1997). *Amos users' guide, Version 3.6.* Mooresville, IN: Scientific Software.

Associates for Research into the Science of Enjoyment (1999). *Home page, http://www.arise.org/.*

Avison, W.R., & Mcalpine, D.D. (1992). Gender differences in symptoms of depression among adolescents. *Journal of Health and Social Behavior, 33,* 77–96.

Bakker, A.B., Buunk, B.P., & Siero, F.W. (1993). Condoomgebruik door heteroseksuelen [Condom use by heterosexuals]. *Gedrag & Gezondheid, 21,* 238–249.

Bandura, A. (1977a). Self-efficacy: Toward a unifying theory of behavioral change. *Psychological Review, 84,* 191–215.

Bandura, A. (1977b). *Social learning theory.* Englewood Cliffs, NJ: Prentice-Hall.

Bandura, A. (1986). *Social foundations of thought and action: A social cognitive theory.* Englewood Cliffs, NJ: Prentice-Hall.

Bandura, A. (1990). Some reflections on reflections. *Psychological Inquiry, 1,* 101–105.

Bandura, A. (1992). On rectifying the comparative anatomy of perceived control: Comments on "Cognates of personal control". *Applied and Preventive Psychology, 1,* 121–126.

Basen-Engquist, K., & Parcel, G.S. (1992). Attitudes, norms, and self-efficacy: A model of adolescents' HIV-related sexual risk behavior. *Health Education Quarterly, 19,* 263–277.

Basen-Engquist, K., Edmundson, E.W., & Parcel, G.S. (1996). Structure of health risk behavior among high school students. *Journal of Consulting and Clinical Psychology, 64,* 764–775.

Bearinger, L.H., & Blum, R.W. (1997). The utility of locus of control for predicting adolescent substance abuse. *Research in Nursing and Health, 20,* 229–245.

Bearman, P.S., Jones, J., & Udry, J.R. (1997). The national longitudinal study of adolescent health: Research design. [WWW document]. URL: *http://www.cpc.unc.edu/ projects/addhealth/design.html.*

Beauchamp, T.L., & Childress, J.F. (1989). *Principles of biomedical ethics.* (3rd ed.). New York: Oxford University Press.

Becker, M.H. (1990). Theoretical models of adherence and strategies of improving adherence. In S.A. Schumaker, E.B. Schron, & J.K. Eckene (Eds.), *Handbook of health behavior change* (pp. 5–43). New York: Springer Publishing Company.

Becker, M.H., Drachman, R.H., & Kirscht, J.P. (1972). Motivations as predictors of health behavior. *Health Services Reports, 87,* 852–862.

Benson, P.L., & Donahue, M.J. (1989). Ten-year trends in at-risk behaviors: A national study of black adolescents. *Journal of Adolescent Research, 4,* 125–139.

Bentler, P.M. (1978). The interdependence of theory, methodology, and empirical data: Causal modeling as an approach to construct validation. In D.B. Kandel (Ed.), *Longitudinal research on drug use: Empirical findings and methodological issues*, (pp. 287–302). New York: John Wiley & Sons.

Bentler, P.M. (1986). *Theory and implementation of EQS: A structural equation program.* Los Angeles: BMDP Statistical Software.

Bentler, P.M., & Speckart, B. (1979). Models of attitude-behavior relations. *Psychological Review, 86,* 452–464.

Bentler, P.M., & Speckart, G. (1981). Attitudes "cause" behaviors: A structural equation analysis. *Journal of Personality and Social Behavior, 40,* 226–238.

Bentler, P.M., & Weeks, D.G. (1980). Linear structural equations with latent variables. *Psychometrika, 45,* 289–307.

Berry, J.W., Poortinga, Y.H., & Pandey, J. (Eds.), (1997). *Handbook of cross-cultural psychology* (2nd ed.), (Vol. 1). Boston: Allyn & Bacon.

Bers, S.A., & Quinlan, D.M. (1992). Perceived competence deficit in anorexia nervosa. *Journal of Abnormal Psychology, 101,* 423–431.

Bijstra, J.O., Van der Kooi, H.P., & Van der Molen, H.T. (1993). Opzet en effecten van een preventieve sociale-vaardigheidstraining voor jong adolescenten *[Design and effect of a preventive social skills training for young adolescents]. Tijdschrijft voor Onderwijsresearch, 186,* 355–368.

Black, N., Boswell, D., Gray, A., Murphy, S., & Popay, J. (Eds.) (1984). *Health and disease: A reader.* London: Open University Press.

Blonz, E.R. (1993). *The really simple, no nonsense nutrition guide.* Berkeley: Conari Press.

Blum, R.W., & Rinehart, P.M. (1997). *Reducing the risk: Connections that make a difference in the lives of youth.* Minneapolis, Minnesota: Division of General Pediatrics and Adolescent Health, University of Minnesota.

Boekaerts, M., & Simons, R.J. (1993). *Leren en instructie [Learning and instruction].* Assen: Dekker & van de Vegt.

Bollen, K.A. (1989). *Structural equations with latent variables.* New York: John Wiley & Sons.

Borkovec, T.D., Robinson, E., Pruzinsky, T., & DePree, J.A. (1983). Preliminary exploration of worry: Some characteristics and processes. *Behavior Research and Therapy, 21,* 9–16.

Botvin, G.J., & Scheier, L.M. (1997). Preventing drug abuse and violence. In D. Wilson, J. R. Rodrigue, & W.C. Taylor (Eds.), *Health promoting and health compromising behaviors among minority adolescents* (pp. 55–86). Washington DC: American Psychological Association.

Boyd, B., & Wandersman, A. (1991). Predicting undergraduate condom use with the Fishbein and Ajzen and the Triandis attitude-behavior models: Implications for public health interventions. *Journal of Applied Social Psychology, 21,* 1810–1830.

Broekman, J.M., Feldmann, H., & Van Haute, P. (Eds.) (1993). *Ziektebeelden* [Images of illness]. Leuven, Belgium: Uitgeverij Peeters.

Brown, L.K., DiClemente, R.J., & Park, T. (1992). Predictors of condom use in sexually active adolescents. *Journal of Adolescent Health, 13,* 651–657.

Brown, L., DiClemente, R., & Reynolds, L. (1991). HIV prevention for adolescents: Utility of the health belief model. *AIDS Education and Prevention, 3,* 50–59.

Brownell, K.D. (1991). Personal responsibility and control over our bodies: When expectations exceed reality. *Health Psychology, 10,* 303–310.

Bush, F.M., Harkings, S.W., Harrington, W.G., & Price, D.D. (1993). Analysis of gender effects on pain perception and symptom presentation in temporomandibular joint pain. *Pain, 53,* 73–80.

Canadian Council for Tobacco Control (1998). Current smoking in Canada among males and females 15–19 year olds 1977–1994. *http://www.cctc.ca/ncth/index.html.*

Cancer Society of New Zealand (1998). Statistics on smoking: Young people and smoking. *http://www.wce.ac.nz/cancer/lifestyles_smokefree/stats.html.*

Caplan, A., Tristram Engelhardt, H.J., & McCartney, J. (Eds.) (1981). *Concepts of health and disease: Interdisciplinary perspectives.* London: Addison-Wesley Publishing Company.

Caprara, V.G., Pastorelli, C., & Weiner, B. (1997). Linkages between causal ascriptions, emotion and behavior. *International Journal of Behavioral Development, 20,* 153–162.

Carr, T., & Schmidt, J.J. (1994). Who's afraid of the...? A survey of eighth graders' concerns. *School Counselor, 42,* 66–72.

Carter, W.B. (1990). Health behavior as a rational process: Theory of reasoned action and multiattribute utility theory. In K. Glanz, F.M. Lewis, & B.K. Rimer (Eds.), *Health behavior and health education: Theory, research, and practice,* (pp.63–91). San Francisco: Jossey Bass.

Centers for Disease Control (1998). Leading causes of mortality and morbidity and contributing behaviors in the United States. *http://www.cdc.gov/nccdphp/dash/ahsumm/ussumm.htm.*

Chapuy, M.C., & Meunier, P.J. (1995). Prevention and treatment of osteoporosis. *Aging (Milano), 7,* 164–173.

Chewning, B., & Van Koningsveld, R. (1998). Predicting adolescents' initiation of intercourse and contraceptive use. *Journal of Applied Social Psychology, 28,* 1245–1285.

Chigier, E., & Nudelman, A. (1994). A cross-cultural approach to health education for immigrants and refugees. *Collegium Antropologicum, 18,* 195–198.

Clark, K., Parr, R., & Castelli, W. (Eds.). (1988). *Evaluation and management of eating disorders: Anorexia, bulimia and obesity.* Champaign, IL: Life Enhancement Publications.

Cluitmans, T., Gouwenberg, N., & Miltenburg, H. (1989). *Gezondheid en leefsituatie van adolescenten in Haarlem.* (2): GGD Zuid-Kennemerland.

Cobb, N.J. (1992). *Adolescence: Continuity, change, and diversity.* Mountain View, CA: Mayfield Publishing Company.

Cobb, N.J. (1998). *Adolescence: Continuity, change and diversity* (3rd ed.). Mountain View, CA: Mayfield Publishing Company.

Cohen, J. (1988). *Statistical power analysis for the behavioral sciences* (2nd ed.). Hillsdale, NJ: Lawrence Erlbaum Associates Inc.

Cohen, R.Y., Brownell, K.D., & Felix, M.R.J. (1990). Age and sex differences in health habits and beliefs of school children. *Health Psychology, 9,* 208–224.

Coleman, J., & Hendry, L. (1990). *The nature of adolescence* (2nd ed.). London: Routledge.

Compas, B.E. (1993). Promoting positive mental health during adolescence. In S.G. Millstein, A.C. Petersen, & E.O. Nightingale (Eds.), *Promoting the health of adolescents: New directions for the twenty-first century* (pp. 159–179). New York: Oxford University Press.

Contento, I.R., & Michela, J.L. (1998). Nutrition and food choice behavior among children and adolescents. In A.J. Goreczny & M. Hersen (Eds.), *Handbook of pediatric and adolescent health psychology.* Boston, MA: Allyn & Bacon.

Cook, T., & Campbell, D. (1979). *Quasi-experimentation: Design and analysis issues for field settings.* Chicago: Rand McNally College Publishing Company.

Cook, T.D., Anson, A.R., & Walchli, S.B. (1993). From causal description to causal explanation: Improving three already good evaluations of adolescent health programs. In S.G. Millstein, A.C. Petersen, & E.O. Nightingale (Eds.), *Promoting the health of adolescents: New directions for the twenty-first century* (pp. 339–374). New York: Oxford University Press.

Costa, F.M., Jessor, R., Fortenberry, J.D., & Donovan, J.E. (1996). Psychosocial conventionality, health orientation, and contraceptive use in adolescence. *Journal of Adolescent Health, 18,* 404–416.

Craig, G.J. (1983). *Human development* (3rd ed.). Englewood Cliffs, NJ: Prentice-Hall.

Crawford, R. (1977). You are dangerous to your health: The ideology of victim blaming. *International Journal of Health Services, 7,* 663–679.

Creswell, J.W. (1998). *Qualitative inquiry and research design: Choosing among five traditions.* Thousand Oaks, CA: Sage Publications.

Crockett, L.J., & Peterson, A.C. (1993). Adolescent development: Health risks and opportunities for health promotion. In S.G. Millstein, A.C. Petersen, & E.O. Nightingale (Eds.), *Promoting the health of adolescents: New directions for the twenty-first century* (pp. 13–37). New York: Oxford University Press.

Cummings, K.M., Becker, M.H., & Maille, M.C. (1980). Bringing the models together: An empirical approach to combining variables used to explain health actions. *Journal of Behavioral Medicine, 3,* 123–145.

Danish, S.J. (1990). Ethical considerations in the design, implementation and evaluation of developmental interventions. In C.B. Fisher & W.W. Tryon (Eds.), *Ethics in applied developmental psychology: Emerging issues in an emerging field.* (pp. 93–112). Norwood, NJ: Ablex Publishing Corp.

De Bourdeaudhuij, I. (1996). Resemblance in healthy behaviors between family members. *Archives of Public Health, 54,* 251–273.

De Bourdeaudhuij, I. (1997a). Family food rules and healthy eating in adolescents. *Journal of Health Psychology, 2,* 45–56.

De Bourdeaudhuij, I. (1997b). Perceived family members' influence on introducing healthy food into the family. *Health Education Research: Theory and Practice, 12,* 77–90.

De Groot, A. (1961). *Methodologie* [Methodology]. 's-Gravenhage, The Netherlands: Uitgeverij Mouton.

De Maio Esteves, M. (1990). Mediators of daily stress and perceived health status in adolescent girls. *Nursing Research, 39,* 360–364.

De Vries, H., & Backbier, E. (1995). Verklaring en verandering van gedrag: Een beschouwing van het transtheroretisch model [Explaining and changing behavior: An examination of the transtheoretical model]. *Tijdschrift Gezondheidsbevordering, 16,* 26–34.

De Vries, H., Dijkstra, M., & Kuhlman, P. (1988). Self-efficacy: The third factor besides attitude and subjective norm as a predictor of behavioural intentions. *Health Education Research: Theory and Practice, 3,* 273–282.

Den Hertog, P. (1992). Determinanten van blessure-preventief gedrag [Determinants of injury-preventive behavior]. *Gedrag en Gezondheid, 20,* 57–72.

Denzin, N.K., & Lincoln, Y.S. (Eds.) (1994). *Handbook of qualitative research.* Thousand Oaks, CA: Sage Publications.

Desmond, S., Price, J.H., & O'Connell, J.K. (1985). Health locus of control and voluntary use of seat belts among high school students. *Perceptual and Motor Skills, 61,* 315–319.

Diekstra, R.F.W., & Methorst, G.J. (1986). De samenleving als verslaver: leefstijl, geestelijke gezondheid en verslavingsrisico bij jongeren [Society as addictive: Lifestyle, psychological well-being, and risk of addiction in adolescents]. *Gedrag & Gezondheid, 14,* 145–152.

Dohrenwend, B.P., & Shrout, P.E. (1985). "Hassles" in the conceptualization and measurement of life stress variables. *American Psychologist, 40,* 780–785.

Donovan, J.E., Jessor, R., & Costa, F.M. (1991). Adolescent health behavior and conventionality-unconventionality: An extension of the problem behavior theory. *Health Psychology, 10,* 52–61.

Donovan, J.E., Jessor, R., & Costa, F.M. (1993). Structure of health-enhancing behavior in adolescence: A latent-variable approach. *Journal of Health and Social Behavior, 34,* 346–362.

Duda, H.L., Smart, A.E., & Tappe, M.L. (1989). Predictors of adherence in the rehabilitation of athletic injuries: An application of personal investment theory. *Journal of Sport and Exercise Psychology, 11,* 367–381.

Eagly, A., & Chaiken, S. (1993). *The psychology of attitudes.* New York: Harcourt Brace Jovanovich College Publishers.

Earls, F. (1993). Health promotion for minority adolescents: Cultural considerations. In S.G. Millstein, A.C. Petersen, & E.O. Nightingale (Eds.), *Promoting the health of adolescents: New directions for the twenty-first century* (pp. 58–72). New York: Oxford University Press.

Edmundson, E., Parcel, G.S., Feldman, H.A., & Elder, J. (1996). The effects of the child and adolescent trial for cardiovascular health upon psychosocial determinants of diet and physical activity behavior. *Preventive Medicine: An International Journal Devoted to Practice and Theory, 25,* 442–454.

Eisen, M., Zellman, G., & McAlister, A. (1992). A health belief model-social learning theory approach to adolescent's fertility control: Findings from a controlled field trial. *Health Education Quarterly, 19,* 249–262.

Eiser, J.R., Eiser, C., Gammage, P., & Morgan, M. (1989). Health locus of control and health beliefs in relation to adolescent smoking. *British Journal of Addiction, 84,* 1059–1065.

Eklind, D. (1978). Understanding the young adolescent. *Adolescence, 13,* 127–134.

Elliot, D.S. (1993). Health-enhancing and health compromising lifestyles. In S.G. Millstein, A.C. Petersen, & E.O. Nightingale (Eds.), *Promoting the health of adolescents: New directions for the twenty-first century* (pp. 119–145). New York: Oxford University Press.

Elmadia, J., & Muskat, K. (1992). *E-nummer wijzer: Hulpstoffen en toevoegsels in onze voedingsmiddelen* [E-number guide: Additives in our food]. Baarn: Tirion.

Elster, J. (1989). Sour grapes—utilitarianism and the genesis of wants. In J. Christman (Ed.), *The inner citadel* (pp. 170–188). New York: Oxford University Press.

Erikson, E.H. (1963). *Childhood and Society.* New York: W.H. Norton & Company.

Fishbein, M. (1967). Attitude and the prediction of behavior. In M. Fishbein (Ed.), *Readings in attitude theory and measurement.* (pp. 477–492). New York: John Wiley & Sons.

Flew, A. (Ed.) (1984). *A dictionary of philosophy.* London: Pan Books.

Flora, J.A., & Maibach, E.W. (1990). Cognitive responses to AIDS information: The effects of issue involvement and message appeal. *Communications Research, 17,* 759–774.

Flynn, B.S., Worden, J.K., Secker-Walker, R., Badger, G., & Geller, B. (1995). Cigarette smoking prevention effects of mass media and school interventions targeted to gender and age groups. *Journal of Health Education, 26,* 45–51.

Fowler, F.J.J. (1993). *Survey research methods* (Vol. 1). Newbury Park, MA: Sage Publications.

Freidson, E. (1971). *The profession of medicine: A study of the sociology of medicine.* New York: Dood & Mead.

Froman, R.D., & Owen, S.V. (1991). High-school students' perceived self-efficacy in physical and mental health. *Journal of Adolescent Research, 6,* 181–196.

Frosch, M. (Ed.) (1995). *Coming of age in America: A multicultural anthology.* New York: The New Press.

Gagné, R.M., & Briggs, L.J. (1979). *Principles of instruction design.* New York: Holt, Rinehart & Winston.

Giblin, P.T. (1992). Psychosocial measures in adolescent health: Reflections of the impact of one's publication on subsequent published research. *Journal of Adolescent Health, 13,* 541–545.

Giblin, P.T., Poland, M.L., & Ager, J.W. (1988). Clinical applications of self-esteem and locus of control to adolescent health. *Journal of Adolescent Health Care, 9,* 1–14.

Gilligan, C. (1988). Adolescent development reconsidered. In C. Gilligan, J. Ward, M. Taylor, & B. Baridge (Eds.), *Mapping the moral domain* (pp. 63–92). Cambridge, MA: Harvard University Press.

Glanz, K., Lewis, F.M., & Rimer, B.K. (Eds.) (1990). *Health behavior and health education: Theory, research, and practice.* San Francisco: Jossey Bass.

Glanz, K., Lewis, F.M., & Rimer, B.K. (Eds.) (1997). *Health behavior and health education: Theory, research, and practice* (2nd ed.). San Francisco: Jossey-Bass Publishers.

Gochman, D.S. (1982). Labels, systems, and motives: Some perspectives for future research and programs. *Health Education Quarterly, 9,* 263–270.

Gochman, D.S. (1988). Health behavior: Plural perspectives In D.S. Gochman (Ed.), *Health behavior: Emerging research perspectives* (pp. 3–17). New York: Plenum Press.

Godin, G., & Shepard, R.J. (1986). Importance of type of attitude to the study of exercise behavior. *Psychological Reports, 58,* 991–1000.

Godin, G., & Shepard, R.J. (1990). Use of attitude-behavior models in exercise promotion. *Sports Medicine, 10,* 103–121.

Goldman, L., & Cook, E.F. (1984). Decline in ischemic heart disease mortality. *Annals of Internal Medicine, 101,* 825–836.

Gore, S., Aseltine, R.H.J., & Colton, M.E. (1992). Social structure, life stress and depressive symptoms in a high school-aged population. *Journal of Health and Social Behavior, 33,* 97–113.

Graham, S. (1992). "Most of the subjects were white and middle class": Trends in published research on African Americans in selected APA journals, 1970–1989. *American Psychologist, 47,* 629–639.

Green, L.W., & Kreuter, M.W. (1991). *Health Promotion Planning: An educational and environmental approach.* Mountain View, CA: Mayfield Publishing Company.

Grimley, D.M., & Lee, P.A. (1997). Condom and other contraceptive use among a random sample of female adolescents: A snapshot in time. *Adolescence, 32,* 771–779.

Grimley, D.M., Riley, G.E., Bellis, J.M., & Prochaska, J. O. (1993). Assessing the stages of change and decision making for contraceptive use for the prevention of pregnancy, sexually transmitted diseases, and acquired immunodeficiency syndrome. *Health Education Quarterly, 20,* 455–470.

Guthrie, B.J., Caldwell, C.H., & Hunter, A.G. (1997). Minority adolescent female health: Strategies for the next millennium. In D. Wilson, J.R. Rodrigue, & W.C. Taylor (Eds.), *Health promoting and health compromising behaviors among minority adolescents* (pp. 153–169). Washington DC: American Psychological Association.

Hacking, I. (1983). *Representing and intervening: Introductory topics in the philosophy of science.* New York: Cambridge University Press.

Haefner, D., & Kirscht, J. (1970). Motivational and behavioral effects of modifying health beliefs. *HSMHA Health Reports, 85,* 478–484.

Haggerty, R.J., Sherrod, L.R., Garmezy, N., & Rutter, M. (Eds.) (1996). *Stress, risk, and resilience in children and adolescents: Processes, mechanisms, and interventions.* Cambridge, UK: Cambridge University Press.

Hamilton, E.M., Whitney, E.N., & Sizer, F.S. (1991). *Nutrition: Concepts and controversies* (5th ed.). St. Paul: West Publishing Company.

Hamilton, S.B., Van Mouwerik, S., Oetting, E.R., Beauvais, F., & Keilin, W.G. (1988). Nuclear war as a source of adolescent worry: Relationships with age, gender, trait emotionality, and drug use. *Journal of Social Psychology, 128,* 745–763.

Havinghurst, R.J. (1972). *Developmental tasks and education.* New York: David McKay.

Hendrikz, A., & De Moor, P. (1982). *Voeding en dieetleer* [Nutrition and diet]. Alphen aan den Rijn, Brussels: Stafleu's Wetenschappelijke Uitgeversmaatschappij B.V.

Hershberger, S. (1994). Specification of equivalent models. In A.Van Eye & C.C. Clogg (Eds.), *Latent variables analysis: Applications for developmental research* (pp. 68–108). Thousand Oaks, CA: Sage Publications.

Heyden, S. (1994). Polyunsaturated and monounsaturated fatty acids in the diet to prevent coronary heart disease via cholesterol reduction. *Annals of Nutrition and Metabolism, 38,* 117–122.

Ho, R. (1992). Cigarette health warnings: The effects of perceived severity, expectancy of occurrence, and self-efficacy on intentions to give up smoking. *Australian Psychologist, 27,* 109–113.

Hochbaum, G.M., Sorenson, J.R., & Loring, K. (1992). Theory in health education practice. *Health Education Quarterly, 19,* 295–313.

Hølund, U. (1990a). Effect of a nutrition education program, "learning by teaching", on adolescents' knowledge and beliefs. *Community Dental Oral Epidemiology, 18,* 61–65.

Hølund, U. (1990b). Promoting change of adolescents' sugar consumption: The "learning by teaching" study. *Health Education Research, 5,* 451–458.

Hoogenboezem, J. (1998). Overleden 10–19 jarigen naar belangrijke doordsoorzaken en geslacht, 1996 [Death of 10–19 year-olds by important causes and gender, 1996]. The Hague: Netherlands Central Bureau for Statistics.

Hoogstraten, J., De Haan, W., & Ter Horst, G. (1985). Stimulating the demand for dental care: An application of Ajzen and Fishbein's theory of reasoned action. *European Journal of Social Psychology, 15,* 401–414.

Hotaling, G.T., Atwell, S.G., & Linsky, A.S. (1978). Adolescent life changes and illness: A comparison of three models. *Journal of Youth and Adolescence, 7,* 393–403.

Huba, G.J., & Melchior, L.A. (1998). A model for adolescent targeted HIV/AIDS services: Conclusions from 10 adolescent-targeted projects funded by the Special Projects of National Significance Program of the Health Resources and Services Administration. *Journal of Adolescent Health, 23,* 11–27.

Hurrelmann, K., Uwe, E., & Weidman, J.C. (1992). Impacts of school pressure, conflict with parents, and career uncertainty on adolescent stress in the Federal Republic of Germany. *International Journal of Adolescence and Youth, 4,* 33–50.

Hurrelmann, K. (1990). Health promotion for adolescents: Preventive and corrective strategies against problem behavior. *Journal of Adolescence, 13,* 231–250.

Hurrelmann, K., & Lösel, F. (1990). Basic issues and problems of health in adolescence. In K. Hurrelmann & F. Lösel (Eds.), *Health hazards in adolescence* (pp. 1–21). Berlin: Walter de Gruyter.

Hurrelmann, K., Engel, U., Holler, B., & Nordlohne, E. (1988). Failure in school, family conflicts, and psychosomatic disorders in adolescence. *Journal of Adolescence, 11,* 237–249.

Illich, I. (1975). *Medical nemesis: The expropriation of health.* London: Calder & Boyers.

Jackson, J.S., & Sellers, S.L. (1997). Psychological, social, and cultural perspectives on minority health in adolescence: A life-course framework. In D. Wilson, J.R. Rodrigue, & W.C. Taylor (Eds.), *Health promoting and health compromising behaviors among minority adolescents* (pp. 29–49). Washington DC: American Psychological Association.

Jakobs, E., Van Schie, E., Van Baaren, K., & Van der Pligt, J. (1993). De perceptie van gezondheidsrisico's door adolescenten: Determinanten van optimisme [The perception of health risks by adolescents: Determinants of optimism]. In B. Verplanken, P.A.M. Van Lange, R.V. Meertens, & F.W. Siero (Eds.), *Toegepaste Sociale Psychologie* (Vol. 7). Delft: Eburon.

Janis, I.L., & Mann, L. (1977). *Decision making: A psychological analysis of conflict, choice, and commitment.* London: Cassell & Collier Macmillan.

Janz, N.K., & Becker, M.H. (1984). The health belief model: A decade later. *Health Education Quarterly, 2,* 1–47.

Jessor, R., & Jessor, S.L. (1977). *Problem behaviour and psychosocial development: A longitudinal study of youth.* New York: Academic Press.

Jessor, R. (1984). Adolescent development and behavioral health. In J.D. Matarazzo, S.M. Weiss, J.A. Herd, & N.E. Miller (Eds.), *Behavioral health: A handbook of health enhancement and disease prevention* (pp. 69–90). New York: Wiley.

Jessor, R. (1991). Risk behavior in adolescence: A psychosocial framework for understanding and action. *Journal of Adolescent Health, 12,* 597–605.

Jessor, R. (1993). Successful adolescent development among youth in high-risk settings. *American Psychologist, 48,* 117–126.

Jessor, R. (Ed.). (1998). *New perspectives on adolescent risk behavior.* Cambridge, UK: Cambridge University Press.

Jessor, R., Colby, A., & Shewder, R.A. (Eds.) (1996). *Ethnography and human development.* Chicago: University of Chicago Press.

Joint Committee on Health Education Terminology (1990). Report of the 1990 joint committee on health education terminology. *Journal of Health Education, 22,* 79–108.

Jöreskog, K. (1990). New developments in LISREL: Analysis of ordinal variables using polychoric correlations and weighted least squares. *Quality and Quantity, 24,* 387–404.

Jöreskog, K.G. (1973). A general method for estimating a linear structural equation system. In A.S. Goldberger & O.D. Duncan (Eds.), *Structural equation models in the social sciences.* New York: Seminar Press/Harcourt Brace.

Jöreskog, K.G., & Sörbom, D. (1986). *LISREL VI.* Mooresville, IN: Scientific Software.

Jöreskog, K., & Sörbom, D. (1993). *Lisrel 8: Structural equation modeling with the SIMPLIS command language.* Chicago: SSI Scientific Software International.

Kanner, A.D., Feldman, S.S., Weinberger, D.A., & Ford, M.E. (1987). Uplifts, hassles, and adaptational outcomes in early adolescence. *Journal of Early Adolescence, 7,* 371–384.

Kaplan, R.M., Sallis, J.F.J., & Patterson, T.L. (1993). *Health and human behavior.* New York: McGraw-Hill.

Kashima, Y., Gallois, C., & McCamish, M. (1993). The theory of reasoned action and cooperative behavior: It takes two to use a condom. *British Journal of Social Psychology, 32,* 227–239.

Kasl, S.V., & Cobb, S. (1966). Health behavior, illness behavior, and sick role behavior. *Archives of Environmental Health, 12,* 246–266, 531–541.

Katch, F.I., & McArdle, W.D. (1993). *Introduction to nutrition, exercise, and health* (4th ed.). Philadelphia: Lea & Febiger.

Kaufman, K.L., Brown, R.T., Graves, K., Henderson, P., & Revolinski, M. (1993). What, me worry? *Clinical Pediatrics, 32,* 8–14.

Kelly, R.B., Zyzanske, S.J., & Almegano, S.A. (1991). Prediction of motivation and behavior change following health promotion: Role of health beliefs, social support, and self-efficacy. *Social Science and Medicine, 32,* 311–320.

Kendall, P.C., & Turk, D.C. (1984). Cognitive-behavioral strategies and health enhancement. In J.D. Matarazzo, S.M. Weiss, J.A. Herd, & N.E. Miller (Eds.), *Behavioral health: A handbook of health enhancement and disease prevention* (pp. 393–405). New York: John Wiley & Sons.

Khan, M.E., Anker, M., Patel, B.C., Barge, S., Sadhwani, J., & Kohle, R. (1991). The use of focus groups in social and behavioral research: Some methodological issues. *World Health Statistics Quarterly, 44,* 145–149.

Kidder, L., & Judd, C. (1986). *Research methods in social relations* (5th ed.). New York: CBS Publishing Japan Ltd.

Kirscht, J. (1983). Preventive health behavior: A review of research and issues. *Health Psychology, 2,* 277–301.

Kirscht, J.P. (1988). The health belief model and predictions of health outcomes. In D.S. Gochman (Ed.), *Health behavior: Emerging research perspectives* (pp. 27–41). New York: Plenum Press.

Klecka, W.R. (1980). *Discriminant analysis.* (Vol. 19). Beverly Hills, CA: Sage Publications.

Klerman, L.V. (1993). The influence of economic factors on health-related behaviors in adolescents. In S.G. Millstein, A.C. Petersen, & E.O. Nightingale (Eds.), *Promoting the health of adolescents: New directions for the twenty-first century* (pp. 38–57). New York: Oxford University Press.

Klingman, A. (1998). Psychological education: Studying adolescents' interests from their own perspective. *Adolescence, 33,* 435–446.

Knight, G.P., & Hill, N.E. (1998). Measurement equivalence in research involving minority adolescents. In V.C. McLoyd & L. Steinberg (Eds.), *Studying minority adolescents: Conceptual, methodological, and theoretical issues.* Mahwah, NJ: Lawrence Erlbaum Associates Inc.

Koelen, M.A. (1988). *Tales of logic: A self-presentational view of health-related behavior.* Unpublished doctoral dissertation, Wageningen University.

Kohlberg, L. (1984). *The psychology of moral reasoning.* New York: Harper & Row.

Kohn, P.M., & Milrose, J.A. (1993). The inventory of high-school students' recent life experiences: A decontaminated measure of adolescent's hassles. *Journal of Youth and Adolescence, 22,* 43–55.

Kok, G., de Vries, H., Mudde, A.N., & Strecher, V.J. (1991). Planned health education and the role of self-efficacy: Dutch research. *Health Education Research: Theory and Practice, 6,* 231–238.

Koops, W. (1990). Adolescentie als thema in de ontwikkelingspsychologie [Adolescence as a theme in developmental psychology]. *Nederlands Tijdschrift voor de Psychologie, 45,* 241–249.

Krause, N.M., & Jay, G.M. (1994). What do global self-related health items measure? *Medical Care, 32,* 930–942.

Krippendorff, K. (1980). *Content analysis: An introduction to its methodology.* Thousand Oaks, CA: Sage Publications.

Kroger, J. (1988). A longitudinal study of ego identity status interview domains. *Journal of Adolescence, 11,* 49–64.

Krueger, R.A. (1994). *Focus groups* (2nd ed.). Thousand Oaks, CA: Sage Publications.

Kulak, C.A., & Bilezikian, J.P. (1998). Osteoporosis: Preventive strategies. *International Journal of Fertility and Women's Medicine, 43,* 56–64.

Lachenbruch, P.A. (1975). *Discriminant analysis.* New York: Hafner.

Laflin, M.T., Moore-Hirschl, S., Weis, D.L., & Hayes, B.E. (1994). Use of the theory of reasoned action to predict drug and alcohol use. *International Journal of the Addictions, 29,* 927–940.

Lamberts, H. (1991). *In het huis van de huisarts: Verslag van het transitieproject* [In the practice of the general practitioner: Report on the transition project]. Lelystad, The Netherlands: Meditekst.

Langer, L.M., & Warheit, G.J. (1992). The pre-adult health decision-making model: Linking decision-making directedness/orientation to adolescent health-related attitudes and behaviors. *Adolescence, 27,* 919–948.

Laraque, D., McLean, D.E., Brown-Peterside, P., & Ashton, D. (1997). Predictors of reported condom use in Central Harlem youth as conceptualized by the health belief model. *Journal of Adolescent Health, 21,* 318–327.

Lau, R.R., Hartman, K.A., & Ware, J.E. (1986). Health as a value: Methodological and theoretical considerations. *Health Psychology, 5,* 25–43.

Lau, R.R., Quadrel, M.J., & Hartman, K.A. (1990). Development and change of young adult's preventive health beliefs and behavior: Influence from parents and peers. *Journal of Health and Social Behavior, 31,* 240–259.

Laura, R.S., & Heaney, S. (1990). *Philosophical foundations of health education.* New York: Routledge.

Lazarus, R.S. (1984). Puzzles in the study of daily hassles. *Journal of Behavioral Medicine, 7,* 375–389.

Lazarus, R.S., DeLongis, A., Folkman, S., & Gruen, R. (1985). Stress and adaptational outcomes: The problem of confounded measures. *American Psychologist, 40,* 770–779.

Levenson, P., Pfefferbaum, B., & Morrow, J. (1987). Disparities in adolescent-physician views of teen health information concerns. *Journal of Adolescent Health Care, 8,* 171–176.

Lewis, D., Belgrave, F.Z., & Scott, R.B. (1990). Patient adherence in minority populations. In S.A. Schumaker, E.B. Schron, & J.K. Ockene (Eds.), *The handbook of health behavior change* (pp. 277–292). New York: Springer Publishing Company.

Lewis, F.M., & Daltroy, L.H. (1990). How causal explanations influence health behavior: Attribution theory. In K. Glanz, F.M. Lewis, & B.K. Rimer (Eds.), *Health behavior and health education: Theory, research, and practice* (pp. 92–114). San Francisco: Jossey Bass.

Liedekerken, P.C., Jonkers, R., De Haes, W.F.M., Kok, G.J., & Saan, J.A.M. (1990). *Effectiveness of health education.* Assen, The Netherlands: Van Gorcum.

Lollis, C.M., Johnson, E.H., & Antoni, M.H. (1997). The efficacy of the health belief model for predicting condom usage and risky sexual practices in university students. *AIDS Education and Prevention, 96,* 551–563.

Mackenbach, J.P. (1992). Socio-economic health differences in the Netherlands: A review of recent empirical findings. *Social Science and Medicine, 34,* 213–226.

Maddux, J.E., & Rogers, R.W. (1983). Protection motivation and self-efficacy: A revised theory of fear appeals and attitude change. *Journal of Experimental Social Psychology, 19,* 469–479.

Maehr, M.L., & Braskamp, L.A. (1986). *The motivation factor: A theory of personal investment.* Lexington, MA: Lexington Press.

Manstead, A.S.R., Proffitt, C., & Smart, J.L. (1983). Predicting and understanding mothers' infant feeding method. *Journal of Personality and Social Psychology, 44,* 657–671.

Marcia, J.E. (1994). The empirical study of ego identity. In H.A. Bosma, T. L.G. Graafsma, H.D. Grotevant, & D.J. de Levita (Eds.), *Identity and development: An interdisciplinary approach* (Sage focus editions, pp. 67–80) Sage Publications, Thousand Oaks, CA.

Marsh, P., Rosser, E., & Harré, R. (1978). *The rules of disorder.* London: Routledge & Kegan Paul.

Masi, L., & Bilezikian, J.P. (1997). Osteoporosis: New hope for the future. *International Journal on Fertility and Women's Medicine, 42,* 245–254.

McGuire, D.P., Mitic, W., & Neumann, B. (1987). Perceived stress in adolescents: What normal teenagers worry about. *Canada's Mental Health, 35,* 2–5.

McGuire, W.J. (1983). A contextualist theory of knowledge: Is implications for innovation and reform in psychological research. *Advances in Experimental Social Psychology, 16,* 1–47.

McGuire, W.J. (1985). Attitudes and attitude change. In G. Lindzey & E. Aronson (Eds.), *Handbook of social psychology* (Vol. 2, pp. 233–246). New York: Lawrence Erlbaum Associates Inc.

McKenzie, J.F., & Lurs, J.L. (1993). *Planning, implementing, and evaluating health promotion programs.* New York: Macmillan Publishing Company.

McLoyd, V.C. (1998). Changing demographics in the American population: Implications for research on minority children and adolescents. In V.C. McLoyd & L. Steinberg (Eds.), *Studying minority adolescents: Conceptual, methodological, and theoretical issues* (pp. 3–28). Mahwah, NJ: Lawrence Erlbaum Associates Inc.

McLoyd, V.C., & Ceballo, R. (1998). Conceptualizing and assessing economic context: Issues in the study of race and child development. In V.C. McLoyd & L. Steinberg (Eds.), *Studying minority adolescents: Conceptual, methodological, and theoretical issues* (pp. 251–278). Mahwah, NJ: Lawrence Erlbaum Associates Inc.

Miles, M.B., & Huberman, A.M. (1994). *Qualitative data analysis: An expanded sourcebook* (2nd. ed.). Thousand Oaks, CA: Sage Publications.

Millstein, S.G. (1989). Adolescent health: Challenges for behavioral scientists. *American Psychologist, 44,* 837–842.

Millstein, S.G. (1993). A view of health from the adolescent's perspective. In S.G. Millstein, A.C. Petersen, & E.O. Nightingale (Eds.), *Promoting the health of adolescents: New directions for the twenty-first century* (pp. 97–118). New York: Oxford University Press.

Millstein, S.G., Petersen, A.C., & Nightingale, E.O. (1993a). Adolescent health promotion: Rationale, goals, and objectives. In S.G. Millstein, A.C. Petersen, & E.O. Nightingale (Eds.), *Promoting the health of adolescents: New directions for the twenty-first century* (pp. 3–12). New York: Oxford University Press.

Millstein, S.G., Petersen, A.C., & Nightingale, E.O. (Eds.) (1993b). *Promoting the health of adolescents: New directions for the twenty-first century.* New York: Oxford University Press.

Moore, C.M. (1987). *Group techniques for idea building* (Vol. 9). Newbury Park, MA: Sage Publications.

Moreillon, J. (1992). Young people's perceptions of health and health care—World Health Organization (WHO) special session: Adolescents in our society. *Journal of Adolescent Health, 13,* 420–430.

Morgan, D.L. (1997). *Focus groups as qualitative research* (2nd ed.) (Vol. 16). Newbury Park, MA: Sage Publications.

Mullen, P., Hersey, J., & Iverson, D. (1987). Health behavior models compared. *Social Science and Medicine, 24,* 973–981.

Murphy, W.G., & Brubaker, R.G. (1990). Effects of a brief theory-based intervention on the practice of testicular self-examination by high school males. *Journal of School Health, 60,* 459–462.

Mutanen, M. (1997). Comparison between dietary monounsaturated and polyunsaturated fatty acids as regards diet-related diseases. *Biomedicine and Pharmacotherapy, 51,* 314–317.

Neimeyer, G.J., Guy, J., & Metzler, W. (1989). Changing attitudes regarding the treatment of disordered eating: An application of the elaboration likelihood model. *Journal of Social and Clinical Psychology, 8,* 70–86.

Netherlands Central Bureau of Statistics (1992). *Netherlands health interview survey.* Den Haag: SDU Publishers.

Newcomb, M.D., & Bentler, P.M. (1987). Self-report methods of assessing health status and health service utilization: A hierarchical confirmatory analysis. *Multivariate Behavioral Research, 22,* 415–436.

Newcomb, M.D., Huba, G.J., & Bentler, P.M. (1981). A multidimensional assessment of stressful life events among adolescents: Derivation and correlates. *Journal of Health and Social Behavior, 22,* 400–415.

Nigg, C.R., & Courneya, K.S. (1998). Transtheoretical model: Examining adolescent exercise behavior. *Journal of Adolescent Health, 22,* 214–224.

Nurmi, J.E., Poole, M.E., & Kalakoski, V. (1994). Age differences in adolescent future-oriented goals, concerns, and related temporal extension in different sociocultural contexts. *Journal of Youth and Adolescence, 23,* 471–487.

Nutricia. (1984). *Nutricia Vademecum.* Zoetermeer: N.V. Nutricia.

Oliver, M. (1997). It is more important to increase the intake of unsaturated fats than to decrease the intake of saturated fats: Evidence from clinical trials relating to ischemic heart disease. *American Journal of Clinical Nutrition, 66* (Suppl. 4), 980S–986S.

Organista, P.B., Chun, K.M., & Marín, G. (Eds.) (1998). *Readings in ethnic psychology.* New York: Routledge.

Orton, G. (1982). A comparative study of children's worries. *Journal of Psychology, 110,* 152–162.

Parcel, G.S. (1976). Skills approach to health education: A framework for integrating cognitive and affective learning. *Journal of School Health, 46,* 403–406.

Parcel, G.S. (1984). Theoretical models for application in school health education research. *Journal of School Health, 54,* 39–49.

Parcel, G.S., Simons-Morton, B.B., & Kolbe, L.J. (1988). Health promotion: Integrating organizational change and student learning strategies. *Health Education Quarterly, 15,* 435–450.

Parr, R.B. (1988). Weight loss: Its effect on normal growth patterns. In K. Clark, R. Parr, & W. Castelli (Eds.), *Evaluation and management of eating disorders: Anorexia, bulimia, and obesity.* (pp. 91–104). Campaign, IL: Life Enhancement Publications.

Pasnick, R.J. (1997). Socioeconomic and cultural factors in the development and use of theory. In K. Glanz, F.M. Lewis, & B.K. Rimer (Eds.), *Health behavior and health education: Theory, research, and practice* (pp. 425–440). San Francisco: Jossey-Bass.

Patten, M.L. (1997). *Understanding research methods.* Los Angeles: Pyrczak Publishing.

Pearce, C.M., & Martin, G. (1993). Locus of control as an indicator of risk for suicidal behavior among adolescents. *Acta Psychiatrica Scandinavica, 88,* 409–414.

Pennebaker, J. (1982). *The psychology of physical symptoms.* New York: Springer-Verlag.

Pennebaker, J.W. (1990). *Opening up: The healing power of confiding in others.* New York: Avon Books.

Perry, C., & Kelder, S.H. (1992). Models for effective prevention. *Journal of Adolescent Health, 13,* 355–363.

Perry, C.L., Baranowski, T., & Parcel, G.S. (1990). How individuals, environments, and health behavior interact: Social learning theory. In K. Glanz, F.M. Lewis, & B.K. Rimer (Eds.), *Health behavior and health education: Theory, research, and practice* (pp. 161–186). San Francisco: Jossey Bass.

Perry, C.L., Kelder, S.H., & Komro, K.A. (1993). The social world of adolescents: Families, peers, schools, and the community. In S.G. Millstein, A.C. Petersen, & E.O. Nightingale (Eds.), *Promoting the health of adolescents: New directions for the twenty-first century* (pp. 73–96). New York: Oxford University Press.

Peterson, C. (1995). Explanatory style and health. In G.M. Buchanan & M.E.P. Seligman (Eds.), *Explanatory style* (pp. 233–246). Hillsdale, NJ: Lawrence Erlbaum Associates Inc.

Peterson, C., & Bossio, L.M. (1991). *Health and optimism.* New York: Free Press.

Petosa, R., & Jackson, K. (1991). Using the health belief model to predict safer sex intentions among adolescents. *Health Education Quarterly, 18,* 463–476.

Petridou, E., Zavitsanos, X., Dessypris, N., Frangakis, C., Mandyla, M., Doxiadis, S., & Trichopoulos, D. (1997). Adolescents in high-risk trajectory: Clustering of risky behavior and the origins of socioeconomic health differentials. *Preventive Medicine, 26,* 215–219.

Petty, R.E., & Cacioppo, J.T. (1981). *Attitudes and persuasion: Classic and contemporary approaches.* Dubuque, IA: WC. Brown Company.

Petty, R.E., & Cacioppo, J.T. (1986). The elaboration likelihood model of persuasion. In L. Berkowitz (Ed.), *Advances in experimental social psychology* (Vol. 19, pp. 123–205). San Diego, CA: Academic Press.

Pipes, P.L., & Trahms, C.M. (1993). *Nutrition in infancy and childhood* (5th ed.). Chicago: Mosby.

Popper, K.R. (1959). *The logic of scientific discovery.* London: Routledge.

Popper, K.R. (1976). *Unended quest: An intellectual autobiography.* Glasgow, UK: Fontana Paperbacks.

Pothmann, R., Frankenberg, S.V., Müller, B., Sartory, G., & Hellmeier, W. (1994). Epidemiology of headache in children and adolescents: Evidence of high prevalence of migraine among girls under 10. *International Journal of Behavioral Medicine, 1,* 76–89.

Prochaska, J.O., & DiClemente, C.C. (1983). Stages and processes of self-change of smoking: Toward an integrative model of change. *Journal of Consulting and Clinical Psychology, 51,* 390–395.

Prochaska, J.O., Velicer, W.F., Rossi, J.D., Goldstein, M.G., Marcus, B.H., Rakowski, W., Fiore, C., Harlow, L.L., Redding, C.A., Rosenbloom, D., & Rossi, S.R. (1994). Stages of change and decisional balance for 12 problem behaviors. *Health Psychology, 13,* 39–46.

Rannie, K., & Craig, D.M.P.H.N. (1997). Adolescent females' attitudes, subjective norms, perceived behavioral control and intentions to use latex condoms. *Public Health Nursing, 14,* 51–57.

Resnick, M.D., Bearman, P.S., Blum, R.W., Bauman, K.E., Harris, K.M., Jones, J., Tabor, J., Beuhring, T., Sieving, R.E., Shew, M., Ireland, M., Bearinger, L., & Udry, J. R. (1997). Protecting adolescents from harm: Findings from the National Longitudinal Study on Adolescent Health. *Journal of the American Medical Association, 278,* 823–832.

Resnick, R.J., & Rozensky, R.H. (Eds.) (1996). *Health psychology through the life span: Practice and research opportunities.* Washington DC: American Psychological Association.

Resnicow, K., Braithwaite, R.L., & Kuo, J. (1997). Interpersonal interventions for minority aadolescents. In D. Wilson, J.R. Rodrigue, & W.C. Taylor (Eds.), *Health promoting and health compromising behaviors among minority adolescents* (pp. 201–223). Washington DC: American Psychological Association.

Resnicow, K., Robinson, T.N., & Frank, E. (1996). Advances and future directions for school-based health promotion research: Commentary on the CATCH intervention trial. *Preventive Medicine: An International Journal Devoted to Practice and Theory, 25,* 378–383.

Riccio-Howe, L. (1991). Health values, locus of control, and cues to action as predictors of adolescent safety belt use. *Journal of Adolescent Health, 12,* 256–262.

Rodin, J. (1986). Aging and health: Effects of the sense of control. *Science, 233,* 1271–1276.

Rogers, R.W. (1975). A protection motivation theory of fear appeals and attitude change. *Journal of Psychology, 91,* 93–114.

Rogers, R.W. (1983). Cognitive and physiological processes in fear appeals and attitude change: A revised theory of protection motivation. In J.T. Cacioppo & R.E. Petty (Eds.), *Social psychophysiology* (pp. 153–176). New York: Guilford Press.

Rosenberg, M.J., & Hovland, C.I. (1960). Cognitive, affective, and behavioral components of attitudes. In C.I. Hovland & M.J. Rosenberg (Eds.), *Attitude organization and change* (pp. 1–14). New Haven, CT: Yale University Press.

Rosenstock, I.M. (1974). Historical origins of the health belief mjodel. *Health Education Monographs, 2,* 328–335.

Rosenstock, R., Strecher, V., & Becker, M. (1988). Social learning theory and the health belief model. *Health Education Quarterly, 15,* 175–183.

Rotter, J.B. (1966). Generalized expectancies for internal versus external control of reinforcements. *Psychological Monographs, 80,* 1–28.

Rouwenhorst, W. (1977). *Leren gezond te zijn?* [Learning to be healthy?]. Alphen aan den Rijn, The Netherlands: Samsom.

Ruwaard, D., & Kramers, P.G.N. (Eds.) (1993). *Volksgezondheid Toekomst Verkenning* [Public health: Exploring the future]. The Hague: Sdu Uitgeverij Plantijnstraat.

Sacks, F.M., & Willet, W.W. (1991). More on chewing the fat: The good fat and the good cholesterol (editorial). *New England Journal of Medicine, 325,* 1740–1742.

Sallis, J.F. (1993). Promoting healthful diet and physical activity. In S.G. Millstein, A.C. Petersen, & E.O. Nightingale (Eds.), *Promoting the health of adolescents: New directions for the twenty-first century* (pp. 209–241). New York: Oxford University Press.

Sandberg, D.E., Rotheram-Borus, M., Bradley, J., & Martin, J. (1988). Methodological issues in assessing AIDS prevention programs. *Journal of Adolescent Research, 3,* 413–418.

Sandler, A.D., Watson, T.E., & Levine, M.D. (1992). A study of the cognitive aspects of sexual decision making in adolescent females. *Journal of Developmental and Behavioral Pediatrics, 13,* 202–207.

Schepers, R.J.M., & Nievaard, A.C. (1990). *Ziekte en zorg, inleiding in de medische sociologie* [Sickness and care, introduction to medical sociology]. Leiden/Antwerpen: Stenfert Kroese Uitgevers.

Schroeder, D.H., & Costa, P.T. (1984). Influence of life event stress on physical illness: Substantive effects or methodological flaws? *Journal of Personality and Social Psychology, 46,* 853–863.

Schwarzer, R., Jerusalem, M., & Kleine, D. (1990). Predicting adolescent health complaints by personality and behaviors. *Psychology and Health, 4,* 233–244.

Scott, C.G., & Ambroson, D.L. (1994). The rocky road to change: Implications for substance abuse programs on college campuses. *Journal of American College Health, 42*, 291–296.

Sears, D.O. (1986). College sophomores in the laboratory: Influences of a narrow data base on psychology's view of human nature. *Journal of Personality and Social Psychology, 51*, 515–530.

Seligman, M.E.P. (Ed.) (1995). *Explanatory style and health*. Hillsdale, NJ: Lawrence Erlbaum Associates Inc.

Seligman, M.E.P., Reivich, K., Jaycox, L., & Gillham, J. (1995). *The optimistic child*. Boston, MA: Houghton Mifflin Co.

Serovich, J.M., & Greene, K. (1997). Predictors of adolescent sexual risk taking behaviors which put them at risk for contracting HIV. *Journal of Youth and Adolescence, 26*, 429–444.

Settertobulte, W., & Kolip, P. (1997). Gender-specific factors in the utilization of medical services during adolescence. *Journal of Adolescence, 20*, 121–132.

Shiloh, S., & Waiser, R. (1991). Adolescents' concepts of health and illness. *International Journal of Adolescent Medicine and Health, 5*, 69–87.

Shope, J.T., Copeland, L.A., Mararg, R., Dielman, T.E., & Butchart, A.T. (1993). Assessment of adolescent refusal skills in an alcohol misuse prevention study. *Health Education Quarterly, 20*, 373–390.

Siebold, D.R., & Roper, R.E. (1979). Psychosocial determinants of health care intentions: Test of the Triandis and Fishbein models. In D. Nimmo (Ed.), *Communication yearbook 3* (pp. 625–643). New Brunswick: Transaction Books.

Silverman, D. (1993). *Interpreting qualitative data: Methods for analysing talk, text, and interaction*. Thousand Oaks, CA: Sage Publications.

Sizer, F., & Whitney, E. (1997). *Nutrition: Concepts and controversies* (7th ed.). Belmont, CA: West/Wadsworth.

Sleek, S. (1998). Behavioral researchers call for more study on human strengths. *American Psychological Association Monitor, 29*, http://www.apa.org/monitor/apr98/human.html.

Sloboda, Z., & David, S. (1997). *Preventing drug use among children and adolescents*. Washington DC: National Institute on Drug Abuse.

Snel, J. (1996). *Geneiten mag! Die dingen die slecht voor ons zijn, zijn vaak heel goed voor ons*. [Enjoy yourself! The things that are bad for us are often very good for us]. Utrecht, The Netherlands: Kosmos Z&K Uitgevers, B.V.

Snyder, T., & Shafer, L. (1996). *Youth Indicators, 1996*. Washington DC: US Department of Education, National Center for Education Statistics.

Society for Public Health Education (1976). *SOPHE's code of ethics*. San Francisco, CA: Society for Public Health Education.

Spruijt, R.J. (1994). Sex differences and the structure of symptom reporting: A latent variable approach. In R.J. Spruijt & K.B. Wabeke, *On temporomandibular joint sounds* (pp. 175–187). Doctoral dissertation, University of Amsterdam.

Spruijt, R.J., & Hoogstraten, J. (1992). Symptom reporting in temporomandibular joint clicking: Some theoretical considerations. *Journal of Craniomandibular Disorders: Facial and Oral Pain, 6*, 213–219.

Spruijt, R.J., & Spruijt-Metz, D. (1994). Aspects of symptom reporting: Age and sex differences. In R.J. Spruijt & K.B. Wabeke, *On temporomandibular joint sounds* (pp. 161–175). Unpublished doctoral dissertation, University of Amsterdam.

Spruijt, R.J., & Wabeke, K.B. (1994). *On temporomandibular joint sounds*. Unpublished doctoral dissertation, University of Amsterdam.

Spruijt-Metz, D. (1995). Personal incentives as determinants of adolescent health behavior: The meaning of behavior. *Health Education Research: Theory and Practice, 10,* 355–364.

Spruijt-Metz, D. (1996). *On everyday health-related behavior in adolescence.* Unpublished doctoral dissertation, Vrije Universiteit Amsterdam.

Spruijt-Metz, D. (1997). Milieubesef en Milieuvriendelijk Gedrag bij Adolescenten: de Theorie van Belangrijke Betekenissen [Adolescents, understanding of environmental questions and environmentally friendly behavior: The theory of salient meanings of behavior], In *Handboek Milieucommunicatie 1997* (pp. D1521–1–D1521–14). Alphen aan den Rijn, The Netherlands: Samson H.D. Tjeenk Willink BV.

Spruijt-Metz, D. (1998a). Gezondheidsgedrag en Gezondheidseducatie bij Adolescenten [Adolescent health behavior and health education]. In J.D. Bosch, H.A. Bosma, R.J. van der Gaag, A.J.J.M. Ruijssenaars, & A. Vyt (Eds.), *Jaarboek Ontwikkelingspsychologie Orthopedagogiek & Kinderpsychiatrie* [Yearbook of developmental psychology, orthopedagogy, and child psychiatry] (pp. 47–75). Houten: Bohn Stafleu.

Spruijt-Metz, D. (1998b). *Salient meanings of health-related behavior.* Paper presented at Out of the Shadow: Visibility and Clarity of Prevention Activities: The 15th Wilhelmina Rouwenhorst lecture, 1997. Trimbos Instituut, Utrecht, The Netherlands.

Spruijt-Metz, D., Hoogstraten, J., & Broekman, J.M. (1994). *Adolescent health and health behavior.* Paper presented at the Thirteenth Biennial Meetings of the ISSBD, Amsterdam, The Netherlands.

Spruijt-Metz, D., & Spruijt, R. (1996). Alledaags gezondhieds- en risicogedrag van adolescenten [Everyday health and risk behaviors in adolescence]. *Gedrag & Gezondheid, 24,* 181–191.

Spruijt-Metz, D., & Spruijt, R. (1997). Worries and health in adolescence: A latent variable approach. *Journal of Youth and Adolescence, 26,* 485–501.

Stacy, A.W., Bentler, P.M., & Flay, B.R. (1994). Attitudes and health behavior in diverse populations: Drunk driving, alcohol use, binge eating, marijuana use, and cigarette use. *Health Psychology, 13,* 72–85.

Stacy, A.W., MacKinnin, D P., & Pentz, M.A. (1993). Generality and specificity in health behavior: Application to warning-label and social influence expectancies. *Journal of Applied Psychology, 78,* 611–627.

Stacy, A.W., Newcomb, M.D., & Bentler, P.M. (1991). Cognitive motivation and problem drug use: A 9 year longitudinal study. *Journal of Abnormal Psychology, 100,* 502–515.

Stanley, B., & Sieber, J.E. (Eds.) (1992). *Social research on children and adolescents: Ethical issues.* Newbury Park, MA: Sage Publications.

Stevens, J. (1992). *Applied multivariate statistics for the social sciences* (2nd ed.). Hillsdale, NJ: Lawrence Erlbaum Associates Inc.

Stewart, D.W., & Shamdasani, P.N. (1990). *Focus groups: Theory and practice.* Newbury Park, MA: Sage Publications.

Strack, R.W., Vincent, M.L., Hussey, J.R., & Kelly, K.M. (1998). Participant characteristics of a nonmandatory school- and community-based sexual risk reduction project. *Family and Community Health, 20,* 63–70.

Strecher, V.J., Kreuter, M., Den Boer, D.J., Kobrin, S., Hospers, H.J., & Skinner, C.S. (1994). The effects of computer-tailored smoking cessation messages in family practice settings. *Journal of Family Practice, 39,* 262–268.

Sturges, J.W., & Rogers, R.W. (1996). Preventive health psychology from a developmental perspective: An extension of protection motivation theory. *Health Psychology, 15,* 158–166.

Swisher, J.D. (1976). Mental health: The core of preventive health education. *Journal of School Health, 56,* 386–391.

Tabachnick, B.G., & Fidell, L.S. (1996). *Using multivariate statistics* (3rd ed.). London: Addison-Wesley.

Tanaka, J.S. (1993). Multifaceted conceptions of fit. In K.A. Bollen & J.S. Long (Eds.), *Testing structural equation models* (pp. 10–39). Newbury Park, MA: Sage Publications.

Tappe, M.K. (1992). The model of personal investment: A theoretical approach for explaining and predicting adolescent health behavior. *Health Education and Research: Theory and Practice, 7,* 277–300.

Tappe, M.K., Duda, J.L., & Menges-Ehrnwald, P. (1990). Personal investment predictors of adolescent motivational orientation toward exercise. *Canadian Journal of Sport Sciences, 15,* 185–192.

Tax, B., Köning-Zahn, C., Heydendael, P.H.J.M., Boerma, L.H., Furer, J.W., Heine, D.J.H.T., Hodiamont, P.P.G., Persoon, J.M.G., & Veling, S.H.J. (1984). Regioproject Nijmegen: Een longitudinaal onderzoek in de bevolking naar ziekte- en hulpzoekgedrag bij somatische klachten, psychiatrische symptomen en psychosociale problemen [Nijmegen regional project: A longitudinal study in the population of illness and help-seeking behaviour for somatic complaints, psychiatric symptoms and psycho-social problems]. *Gezondheid & Samenleving, 5,* 38–45.

Taylor, S.E. (1986). *Health psychology.* New York: Random House.

Taylor, W.C., Beech, B.M., & Cummings, S.S. (1997). Increasing physical activity levels among youth: A public health challenge. In D. Wilson, J.R. Rodrigue, & W.C. Taylor (Eds.), *Health promoting and health compromising behaviors among minority adolescents* (pp. 107–128). Washington DC: American Psychological Association.

Telama, R., Yang, X., Laasko, L., & Viikari, J. (1997). Physical activity in childhood and adolescence as predictor of physical activity in young adulthood. *American Journal of Preventive Medicine, 13,* 317–323.

Terre, L., Ghiselli, W., Taloney, L., & DeSouza, E. (1992). Demographics, affect, and adolescents' health behaviors. *Adolescence, 27,* 13–24.

Thomas, L. (1979). *The Medusa and the snail.* New York: Bantum.

Tones, K., & Tilford, S. (1994). *Health education: Effectiveness, efficiency and equity* (2nd ed.). London: Chapman & Hall.

Triandis, H.C. (1977). *Interpersonal behavior.* Monterey, CA: Brook/Cole.

Tynjala, J., Kannas, L., & Valimaa, R. (1993). How young Europeans sleep. *Health Education Research, 8,* 69–80.

US Department of Health and Human Services (1980). *Promoting health/preventing disease: Objectives for the nation.* Washington, DC: US Government Printing Office.

US Department of Health and Human Services (1995). *Healthy people review: 1994* (DHHS publication no. PHS 95–12561). Washington DC: US Government Printing Office.

Valois, P., Desharnais, R., & Godin, G. (1988). A comparison of the Fishbein and Ajzen and the Triandis attitudinal models for the prediction of exercise intention and behavior. *Journal of Behavioral Medicine, 11,* 459–472.

Van Ameijden, E.J., Van den Hoek, A.J.A.R., Van Haastrecht, H.H., & Coutinho, R.A. (1994). Trends in sexual behavior and the incidence of sexually transmitted diseases and HIV among drug-using prostitutes, Amsterdam 1986–1992. *AIDS, 8,* 213–221.

Van Asselt, A., & Lanphen, W.E.N. (1990). *Gezondheid en leefstijl van jongeren in Flevoland in 1990* [Health and life-style of young people in Flevoland]. (2D): GGD Flevoland.

Van den Putte, B. (1993). *On the theory of reasoned action.* Unpublished doctoral dissertation, University of Amsterdam.

Van der Kamp, L.J.T., Bijleveld, C.C.J.H., Van der Burg, E., Van der Kloot, W. A., Van der Leeden, R., & Mooijaart, A. (1992). *Longitudinal data analysis for the behavioral sciences.* University of Leiden, Department of Psychometrics and Research Methodology, Faculty of Social Sciences.

Van Vliet, K. (1992). *Symptoomwaarneming bij vrouwen met medisch onverklaarde gynaecologische klachten* [Symptom perception in women with unexplained gynaecological complaints]. Unpublished doctoral thesis, University of Amsterdam.

Velicer, W.F., DiClemente, C.C., Rossi, J.S., & Prochaska, J.O. (1990). Relapse situations and self-efficacy: An integrative model. *Addictive Behaviors, 15,* 271–283.

Velicer, W.F., Prochaska, J.O., Fava, J.L., Norman, G.J., & Redding, C.A. (1998). Smoking cessation and stress management: Applications of the transtheoretical model of behavior change. *Homeostasis in Health and Disease, 38,* 216–233.

Verhips, G.H. (1993). *Child dental health and ethnicity in the Netherlands.* Unpublished doctoral dissertation, University of Amsterdam.

Vervaet, M., Van Heeringen, C., & Jannes, C. (1998). Weight concerns and eating patterns in schoolboys and girls. *Eating Disorders: The Journal of Treatment and Prevention, 6,* 41–50.

Viera, A., Pollock, J., & Golez, F. (1998). *Reading educational research* (3rd ed.). New Jersey: Merrill, Prentice Hall.

Viet, L., Baltissen, A., & Syperda, O. (1995). *Onderzoek naar leefgewoonten van jongeren in de regio Ijssel-Vecht* [Study of the lifestyles of the youth in the region of Ijssel-Vecht]. GGD Zuid Kennemerland.

Vobecky, J.S., Vobecky, J., & Normand, L. (1995). Risk and benefit of low fat intake in childhood. *Annals of Nutrition and Metabolism, 39,* 124–33.

Voedingsraad (1986). *Advies richtlijnen goede voeding* [Advice concerning guidelines for good nutrition]. The Hague, The Netherlands: Voedingsraad.

Voorlichting voor de Voeding (1993). *Zo eet Nederland, 1992* [This is how Holland eats, 1992]. Den Haag: Ministry of health, welfare, and culture, Ministry of agriculture, natural resources and fishing.

Wadden, T.A., Brown, G., Foster, G.D., & Linowitz, J.R. (1991). Salience of weight-related worries in adolescent males and females. *International Journal of Eating Disorders, 10,* 407–414.

Waldron, I. (1983). Sex differences in illness incidence, prognosis and mortality: Issues and evidence. *Social Science and Medicine, 17,* 1107–1123.

Wallander, J., & Siegel, L.J. (Eds.). (1995). *Adolescent health problems.* New York: Guilford Press.

Wang, M.Q., Fitzhugh, E., Eddy, J.M., & Westerfield, R. (1996). Attitudes and beliefs of adolescent experimental smokers: A smoking prevention perspective. *Journal of Alcohol and Drug Education, 41,* 1–12.

Watson, D., & Pennebaker, J.W. (1989). Health complaints, stress, and distress: Exploring the central role of negative affectivity. *Psychological Review, 96,* 234–254.

Weiner, B. (1995). *Inferences of responsibility: A foundation for a theory of social conduct.* New York: Guilford Press.

Weiss, B., Weiss, J.R., Politano, M., & Carey, M. (1991). Developmental differences in the factor structure of the Children's Depression Inventory. *Psychological Assessment, 3,* 38–45.

Weiss, R.S. (1994). *Learning from strangers: The art and method of qualitative interview studies.* New York: The Free Press.

West, J. (1999). *Structural equation models.* http://www.gsm.uci.edu/~joelwest/SEM/index.html.

West, K., DuRant, R., & Pendergrast, R. (1993). An experimental test of adolescents' compliance with dental appointments. *Journal of Adolescent Health, 14,* 384–389.

Whitehead, W.E. (1994). Assessing the effects of stress on physical symptoms. *Health Psychology, 13,* 99–102.

Wilson, D.K., Nicholson, S.C., & Krishnamoorthy, J. S. (1997a). The role of diet in minority adolescent health promotion. In D. Wilson, J.R. Rodrigue, & W.C. Taylor (Eds.), *Health promoting and health compromising behaviors among minority adolescents* (pp. 129–151). Washington DC: American Psychological Association.

Wilson, D., Rodrigue, J.R., & Taylor, W.C. (Eds.) (1997b). *Health promoting and health compromising behaviors among minority adolescents.* Washington DC: American Psychological Association.

Worden, J.K., Flynn, B.S., Geller, B.N., Chen, M., Shelton, L., Secker-Walker, W., Solomon, D., Solomon, L., Couchey, S., & Costanza, M. (1988). Development of a smoking prevention mass media program using diagnostic and formative research. *Preventive Medicine, 17,* 531–558.

World Health Organization (1986). *Ottawa charter for health promotion.* Paper presented at the First International Conference in Health Promotion.

World Health Organization (1998). *World Health Report 1998: Life in the 21st century—a vision for all.* Geneva: WHO.

Wu, K.K., & Lam, D.J. (1993). The relationship between daily stress and health: Replicating and extending previous findings. *Psychology and Health, 8,* 329–344.

Yarcheski, A., Mahon, M., & Yarcheski, T. (1997). Alternate models of positive health practices in adolescents. *Nursing Research, 46,* 85–92.

Zola, I.K. (1966). Culture and symptoms: An analysis of peoples presenting complaints. *American Sociological Review, 5,* 141–155.

Indexes

Author Index

Subject Index

For Product Safety Concerns and Information please contact our EU
representative GPSR@taylorandfrancis.com Taylor & Francis Verlag GmbH,
Kaufingerstraße 24, 80331 München, Germany

Printed and bound by CPI Group (UK) Ltd, Croydon, CR0 4YY
08/06/2025
01897007-0009